"Eastern medical traditions place great emphasis of healthy digestion to overall health and well being. In the modern world, it seems more people than ever are suffering from allergies or intolerance to more and more foods. While there are aisles and piles of digestive aids we can turn to for symptom management, they generally do not address root causes of digestive disorders. Nadya Andreeva helps us explore possible root causes and how to improve our health through improving our 'bellies'."

DR. CLAUDIA WELCH

DOM, author of *Balance Your Hormones, Balance Your Life: Achieving Optimal Health and Wellness through Ayurveda, Chinese Medicine, and Western Science*

"I could not be more in line with Nadya Andreeva's message in her book, *Happy Belly*. Indeed, the state of the gut is the state of the body at large. Excellent digestion is the foundation of vitality and beauty. Whether you want more energy or a flat stomach (or both), *Happy Belly* is a must read!"

NATALIA ROSE

Certified Nutritionist, author of 8 books including *The Raw Food Detox Diet, Raw Food Life Force Energy, Detox 4 Women, Emotional Eating S.O.S.*; founder of Detox The World www.detoxtheworld.com

"Finally an easy way to keep a healthy diet. *Happy Belly* is easy to understand and chock full of practical information. A must read for any yogi!"

ELLEN VERBEEK

Editor, *Yoga Journal*, Russia

"Nadya has successfully used her own story, combined with the ancient wisdom of Ayurveda, to offer practical solutions to women challenged by digestive issues. Through its body, mind, and spirit approach, *Happy Belly* will allow many women to skillfully handle what life asks them to digest."

ERIC GRASSER MD
Cay Integrative Medicine & Ayurveda
www.drgrasser.com

"The first step in healing yourself is healing your gut. Digestion is the cornerstone of health. If you or someone you know wants to achieve optimal health and get a flat stomach, too—this book is a must read."

ALEXANDRA JAMIESON
Certified Holistic Health Counselor, author of
The Great American Detox Diet, Vegan Cooking for Dummies,
and *Living Vegan for Dummies*
www.alexandrajamieson.com

"This thoughtful little book steers us back to the fundamental principle that eating mindfully is every bit as important as eating healthfully."

MYRA KORNFELD
Author of *The Healthy Hedonist Holidays, A Year of Multi-Cultural Vegetarian-Friendly Holiday Feasts, The Healthy Hedonist,* and *The Voluptuous Vegan*; head chef and content manager of MyFoodMyHealth.com; teacher at The Natural Gourmet School of Health and Culinary Arts and the Institute of Culinary Education in New York City

"*Happy Belly* will help you to understand the language of your body and help you move toward optimal health. Nadya's approachable blend of modern research, with healthy food and lifestyle choices, will help any woman create a vibrant, radiant body from the inside out."

MARY O'MALLEY

Empowerment coach and author of *The Gift of Our Compulsions*

"I suffered from digestive issues for years, and it was only by listening to the language of my own body, as Nadya suggests, that I was able to overcome them. Nadya is the ultimate guide in helping you understand how you may be standing in your own way to optimal digestive health."

ISABEL FOXEN DUKE

Emotional eating coach: www.isabelfoxenduke.com

"While food is an important aspect of having a healthy body and a flat stomach, our habits around food and eating play a huge role. Nadya brings a new kind of awareness to the behaviors that can help create an efficient digestion and help our body heal. *Happy Belly* provides guidance, ushering the reader on a path to greater wellness. Nadya's insights will shine a ray of light to many who are confused with overwhelming information on food."

JOVANKA CIARES

Author, speaker, wellness expert, producer

"I will happily recommend *Happy Belly* to my clients and students for them to gain an integrated, practical action guide to improve their digestion, absorption, and overall health. For anyone interested in the holistic wisdom ayurveda can offer your gut, let Nadya unpack it for you in her loving, unpretentious manner."

CATE STILLMAN
Founder of www.yogahealer.com
Yoga and ayurveda teacher

"Nadya makes digestive health approachable and simple to understand. *Happy Belly* will help you to make friends with your body and get it on a completely new level."

NITIKA CHOPRA
Talk Show Host; founder of YourBellaLife.com

"Nadya Andreeva radiates the health and the vibrant beauty to which every woman wants access—and can now have through her teachings. With a deep understanding of the relationship between body and mind, *Happy Belly* is a road map to better mind-body relationship, digestion, and self-understanding."

DR. TRACY THOMAS
MA, Ph.D., Licensed Psychologist and Coach

HAPPY BELLY

NADYA ANDREEVA

HAPPY BELLY

a woman's guide to feeling
vibrant, light, and balanced

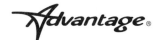

Published by Advantage, Charleston, South Carolina.
Member of Advantage Media Group.

ADVANTAGE is a registered trademark and the Advantage colophon is a trademark of Advantage Media Group, Inc.

Printed in the United States of America.

ISBN: 978-159932-417-3
LCCN: 2013954631

This publication is designed to provide accurate and authoritative information in regard to the subject matter covered. It is sold with the understanding that the publisher is not engaged in rendering legal, accounting, or other professional services. If legal advice or other expert assistance is required, the services of a competent professional person should be sought.

Advantage Media Group is proud to be a part of the Tree Neutral® program. Tree Neutral offsets the number of trees consumed in the production and printing of this book by taking proactive steps such as planting trees in direct proportion to the number of trees used to print books. To learn more about Tree Neutral, please visit **www.treeneutral.com**. To learn more about Advantage's commitment to being a responsible steward of the environment, please visit **www.advantagefamily.com/green**

TreeNeutral

Advantage Media Group is a publisher of business, self-improvement, and professional development books and online learning. We help entrepreneurs, business leaders, and professionals share their Stories, Passion, and Knowledge to help others Learn & Grow. Do you have a manuscript or book idea that you would like us to consider for publishing? Please visit **advantagefamily.com** or call **1.866.775.1696.**

Some of the material in this book has previously appeared online under my name in *Mind Body Green, Holistic Times, Modern Hippie Mag, Chalk Board Magazine,* and in my own website *Spinach and Yoga.*

Thank you to Alex for helping me bring this book into the world. Without your support and encouragement I would never have believed in myself enough to accomplish this.

Thank you to my parents for supporting me in everything that I ever wanted to do and for bringing me up on the best food they knew and could afford. Thank you for bringing me up with a belief in the healing power of the human mind, whole foods, and herbs. I use what you taught me every day and I am forever grateful to you.

acknowledgements

I am grateful to have had wonderful people helping me in the process of writing. A huge thank you to my friend and inspiration Dana James, who contributed advice, encouragement, and a wonderful chapter on food sensitivities.

Thank you to Claudia Welch, Robin Lee, and Lissa Rankin for inspiration, wonderful books that were great resources, and for spreading the message of healing in this world.

I am grateful to Sue Ellen for reviewing the manuscript, advising me, and keeping me motivated. You had a lot more influence than you realize!

Thank you to all who shared their healing stories and to all my clients who taught me about individualized approaches to health, the power of intention, and commitment to feeling great no matter what.

Thank you to my editor, Brooke White, who provided the first girl's opinion, for helping me restructure the book into the most reader-friendly format.

Without all of you, the book would be incomplete.

author's note

This book is designed to provide a new perspective on relating to one's body and food and choosing the best personalized diet for your body. It is sold with the understanding that the publisher and author are not engaged in rendering medical, health, or other professional services. If medical or other expert assistance is required, the services of a competent professional should be sought.

It is not the purpose of this book to reprint all the information that is otherwise available on the topics of health, digestion, and ayurveda. It is meant to complement, amplify, and supplement other existing books. You are urged to read all the available material, learn as much as possible about nutrition, digestion, and ayurveda and tailor the information to your individual needs.

For more information, see the many resources available online and mentioned throughout the book.

The purpose of this manual is to educate and inspire. The author and Advantage Media Group shall have neither liability nor responsibility to any person or entity with respect to any loss or damage caused, or alleged to have been caused, directly or indirectly, by the information contained in this book.

foreword

What we affectionately call the "gut" can serve us well. This internal organ that processes all the food we eat has often been referred to as another brain. The gut knows what is good for it. And when we slip up, it lets us know in no uncertain terms. When we become mindful of how this all works, and how the gut works for us, we can use this information to better take care of ourselves.

The body is constantly giving us signals that the mind does not always pick up on. It takes practice to tune into the body, because the mind speaks so loudly. The mind just wants what it wants, while the gut often suffers the consequences.

You've probably heard the term "gut instinct" bandied about. There is a lot to this. When we listen to that instinct, we are most likely pointing ourselves in the best direction. We have choices to make all the time, from the foods we eat, to the media we follow, to the places we go. Unfortunately, we're all so busy, so distracted, that we aren't always paying attention to our digestion.

Of those who suffer from irritable bowel syndrome (IBS), 65 percent are female. A lot of women are so "on the go" that they have no time to "go" and suffer from chronic constipation. Did you know that you could die from constipation? It's true. We have gotten ourselves so out of balance by eating poorly and popping laxatives that it affects every aspect of our lives. We're feeling miserable, and it all goes back to our digestion. It's time for everyone, and particularly women, to learn to take care of themselves and to get into habits that keep us healthy and strong and feeling great!

The first time I spoke with Nadya Andreeva, I had a really good feeling that this woman had big gifts to offer the world. I was impressed with her online show, her blog, and the messages she sends out through social media. Nadya is bright and beautiful and filled with warm energy and enthusiasm. She exudes compassion and understanding—and she has a passion for ayurveda, as I do. She is a wonderful example of the benefits of living an ayurvedic lifestyle.

When I read Nadya's book, *Happy Belly*, I knew that my initial gut instinct about her was right on. This book is filled with great information that we all need to know and use every single day so that we can have a happy, healthy belly!

Ayurveda dates back more than 5,000 years. It teaches us the art of living in harmony with nature. In our modern society, with our fast-food culture and smart-phone addictions, we're so programmed into reaching for whatever is convenient, hardly taking our attention away from the screens. We have gotten away from nature, and our own nature, sacrificing our digestion all along the way. When we get back to the basics, and start showing the body just how much it is loved and cared for, our body loves us right back. Stress eases, weight falls off, health improves, and happiness reigns supreme!

Ayurveda explains that we're not just what we eat. Rather, we are what we digest. Nadya explains very clearly the steps we can take to maximize our digestion for optimal health. Read this book and mentally digest everything in it. Then go out and take Nadya's advice. Your belly will thank you.

LISSA COFFEY

Lifestyle, wellness, and relationship expert Host/Producer at
http://www.coffeytalk.com

Author: *What's Your Dosha, Baby?*
http://www.whatsyourdosha.com

Author: *What's Your Dharma?*
http://www.whatsyourdharma.com

contents

· ·

introduction

Welcome to the beginning pages of *Happy Belly*, your road map to making friends with your body, ending your battle with bloating, constipation, and getting your flatter stomach back.

Have you heard the statement "You are what you eat"? Most of us hear it hundreds of times throughout our lives. Various nutrition experts, doctors, our parents, and maybe a health-obsessed foodie at work repeat this statement like a magic curse.

Whether you believe this statement or not, you are about to be surprised.

This statement is not true! *You are not what you eat.* You are a lot more complicated than that. But even if we were to dramatically simplify the human body to a food equation, it would be:

You are what you digest, the nutrients you assimilate, and the waste that you eliminate.

Basically, you can eat the cleanest most organic foods and still feel constipated, bloated, and fatigued if you are not digesting them well and not eliminating all the leftover material.

The body is an amazing vehicle that allows us to experience life and to enjoy many pleasures. When basic physiological functions work the way nature intended, we live in blissful ignorance of nature's genius. However, when things go wrong and our body works at a less than perfect rate, we are forced to recognize the intricate design of our internal systems. Healthy digestion is an essential element in achieving a fulfilling, high-quality life.

Our body is constantly renewing and building new cells. Skin, bones, liver, blood—our entire body renews itself on a daily basis. New cells are being built out of the nutrients that we get from the food. If the food that we eat is not nutritious, if our body is not absorbing the nutrients or not eliminating the waste, the new cells cannot be healthy.

A healthy belly digests food well and makes the entire body feel energized, light, and happy.

Unfortunately, many of us are way too familiar with the way an unhappy belly feels and looks: bloated, gassy, heavy, sluggish, and irregular. To be more exact, 60 to 70 million people in the United States are affected by all kinds of digestive diseases, according to the National Institutes of Health.[1] An incredible 63 million people are chronically constipated, as reported in 2000.[2] Chronic constipation costs a staggering $141.8 billion (2004) per year in medical expenses. Worldwide, irritable bowel syndrome (IBS) affects between 9 and 20 percent of the population, making it the most common gastrointestinal disorder. It is estimated that some 35 million Americans suffer from IBS. In the United States alone there are between 2.4 million and 3.5 million annual physician visits for IBS. Women are more likely to suffer from IBS and account for 60 to 65 percent of those diagnosed. However, many others put up with the digestive unease and never get diagnosed.

One in every three people experiences some sort of digestive discomfort throughout the day. It can range from embarrassing gas, constipation, bloating, acid reflux, heartburn, and burping to diarrhea or heaviness after meals.

Digestion affects our immune system, mood, hormones, skin, body odor, and sex drive. When the digestive system is not functioning well, the effects spread to the entire body. The energy level goes down, mental fog and poor focus become regular companions, bad moods or even depression and anxiety can emerge, skin is negatively affected, being social can be a challenge, and the stomach becomes a focus of an angry, self-criticizing monologue toward the body.

If you want a beautiful, healthy, and strong body, you owe it to yourself to understand how your digestion functions and how to keep it in a thriving, optimal state.

WHAT TO EXPECT FROM THIS BOOK

This book is a guide for women who are looking to feel light, easy, and comfortable in their body. It is not meant to be a scientific encyclopedia that you need a dictionary to understand, but is instead written more like a conversation that I would have with a wellness coaching client or a close friend.

This book will teach you how to approach your food, how to be more in tune with your body, and how to stop feeling overwhelmed by all the conflicting information out there. It is not just a set of rules to follow or foods to eat in order to prevent bloating, promote regularity, and avoid painful cramps. I hope that this book will inspire and empower you to think differently about what you put into your body and how you do it. I hope it will also change the way you look at the nutrition articles and the way you think about nourishing your body.

Happy Belly will be helpful in understanding the underlying causes of digestive unease, including things that doctors may not be even considering, let alone telling you—things such as stress, negative thought patterns, and destructive emotions and behaviors around food.

The main take-aways are the principles that can be applied to daily eating and living in general. While this book is about healing the digestive system, the practices you will discover will be healing to your body and your relationship with food in general.

I believe that every woman should feel empowered to take the responsibility for her own health, to dive into exploration, trial and error, and to learn from her body. I also believe that the body carries centuries' worth of wisdom that we can learn to access and understand if we slow down and listen. Your body wants to be healthy and light and to feel amazing. This book is about allowing body wisdom to emerge and supporting the healing process by improving the mind-body connection.

The book consists of four parts. In Part 1 we will talk about why digestion is the cornerstone of good health and the reasons that so many of us suffer from poor digestion, including bloating and constipation. You will get to assess your digestion through a questionnaire and get to know your body better through a tongue diagnosis and examining your poop (yep, gotta look there too!).

In Part 2 you will learn what stands behind digestive unease, bloating, fatigue, constipation, and accompanying feelings of guilt and self-loathing. I will show you how certain eating behaviors can trigger uncomfortable digestive symptoms. Dana James, a certified nutritionist, will tell you the ins and outs of food sensitivities, and you will understand the effect that morning Joe, antibiotics, and antacid drugs have on your tummy.

Part 3 is your Happy Belly road map! We will break down the physical and emotional aspects of healing digestion, getting a flat stomach back, and reconnecting with the body. You will learn about the fascinating ancient science of ayurveda and the amazing benefits it can offer you in today's modern world. You will get to appreciate your body's unique needs and learn to make decisions about which diet to follow to feel your best. We will talk about healthy eating habits, nourishing and easy-to-digest food, the healing effects of deep relaxation, soothing herbal teas, and ways to let go of emotional eating. You will learn the intricacies of the Happy Belly approach to exercise in order to improve regularity and blood circulation in your digestive system.

In Part 4 we will go over the guidelines to feel comfortable and not sabotage your health at social occasions. We will also get into specifics of managing constipation, bloating, and gas, and discuss a simple way to detox. You will learn effective natural remedies that will help to balance your digestion and regain health in these specific cases.

THIS BOOK IS FOR YOU IF

- you feel confused about which nutrition approach/diet is best to follow.

- your stomach gets bloated easily and makes you look pregnant.

- you are afraid of certain foods because of the way they make your stomach feel.

- you dread going out to new restaurants or traveling because you are afraid that you won't find anything good to eat.

- you want to understand what triggers bloating, irregularity, gas, and cramps.

- you want to feel sexy and at ease in your body, not puffy and bloated.

- you want to have a regular bowel movement every morning without effort or straining.

- you feel that your obsession with food is negatively affecting your relationships.

- food is always on your mind, and you would rather spend time thinking about other more creative things.

- you are tired of choosing clothing based on whether it covers your bloated stomach and you would much rather feel sexy in your outfits.

- you want to heal in a holistic natural way; you know that there is more than just food to the total health equation.

- you believe that your body is unique and that you deserve a unique approach.

THIS BOOK IS NOT FOR YOU IF

- you want a quick fix, a pill that will make all the symptoms go away without changing any behaviors and eating patterns.

- you hope that someone can make decisions for you when it comes to food.

- you like restricting and controlling your body.

- you hate to experiment.

- you believe that doctors are responsible for keeping you healthy, that it is their job and you want nothing to do with it.

- you are at peace with the way you feel, and there is nothing that could be improved in your energy levels, digestion, or mood.

This book can be helpful as a lifestyle improvement tool for people with serious gastrointestinal issues who are under the care of a gastroenterologist. It is not in any case a substitute for medication or doctor's care.

NOTE OF CAUTION

We, as humans, crave immediate improvement. Our dream is to find a pill or a person who can make us perfectly healthy, vibrant, and happy overnight. That's why we are so tempted by the advertisements of supplements that claim to work almost immediately without us having to change our behavior. Accepting the fact that no long-term change can occur without an internal shift in beliefs that lead to the change in behaviors can be a bit painful. It comes with resistance.

I will let you in on a secret. When I started teaching, I understood that it is almost pointless to teach people anything. The best teachers don't just share information; they help students realize the truth themselves. This way new information becomes students' own wisdom because they come to it through experiencing it in their body and formulating it in their own words.

This is particularly true with digestion. Throughout the book I will encourage you to try certain things and experiment. Whether they work for your body or not only you can tell. It is your journey of learning and finding your wisdom.

Progress can happen a lot faster when we have some guidance in terms of what things to try and what results to look for. This is the only role I could ever hope for: to be your guide.

So the note of caution is that I am not offering a quick solution or a list of supplements that will "fix" things. I am offering guidance and sharing what has become my wisdom through experience in the hope of helping you to start your own journey of experimenting and learning. Most likely, it will be a lifelong journey because we have to nourish our body every day, and with the changes in the environment, we will have to learn to adapt continuously. The best we can do is to create a strong connection between our body and ourselves and to use our body's wisdom on a daily basis to make choices in any environment.

Don't be intimidated by the long journey. It can be fun: you will learn amazing things about yourself and your body; you will find new friends; and at some point we all come back to help and inspire others. Enjoy your ride!

part one

DIGESTION—
THE CORNERSTONE
OF HEALTH

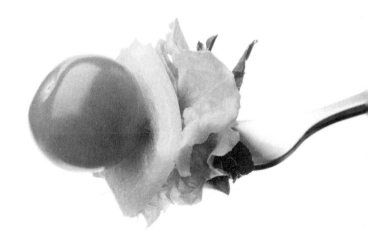

chapter 1

ENERGY, MOOD, CONFIDENCE, IMMUNITY AND GUT CONNECTION

There is no happy life without a healthy gut. The gastrointestinal (GI) tract is an essential part of our physiology, and its health to a large extent determines our health and happiness.

Digestion is considered to be a cornerstone of health by holistic medicine practitioners, including traditional Chinese medicine and ayurveda, the ancient Indian science of health, and most integrative medicine doctors. No matter how much high-quality organic produce you eat, if you can't digest it and assimilate the nutrients while efficiently eliminating the waste, your body will have a hard time building healthy cells, neurotransmitters, and good blood. Gut health has been linked to our learning capacity and memory, depression and anxiety, bone formation, neurological functions, and much more.

Dr. Alexandro Junger, the author of *Clean*[3] and *Clean Gut*,[4] explains the importance of gut health very simply and powerfully: before chronic disease, there is inflammation, but before inflammation comes gut dysfunction. Inflammation in the gut is at the root of almost all, if not all, chronic disease. Dr. Junger points out that heart disease, cancer, diabetes, insomnia, asthma, depression, autoimmune disorders, and arthritis can all be traced back to the injured and irritated gut. He also attributes tiredness, aches and pains, allergies, mood swings, lack of libido, bad breath, body odor, and eczema to gut dysfunction.

The efficiency of digestion determines the strength of your life force in a big way. Your physical body and your emotional body are interconnected. If your physical body is deprived of nutrients and exhausted after years of internal struggle with difficult-to-digest foods, it will project accordingly in your emotions and mood. If you want to live a fulfilling, happy life in which you enjoy your body and all the pleasures it allows you to experience, you need to have a healthy digestion.

Many books have been written about the connection between digestive health and our brain function. Dr. Mark Hyman, in his book *Ultramind Solution*,[5] says that if mental and emotional problems are long standing and have no apparent reason other than regular life's ups and downs, leaky gut syndrome, food sensitivities, or heavy metals in the digestive tract can be the reason.

Health of the gut has also been linked to autism, learning disabilities, sleep disorders, and Parkinson's.[6] Researchers from McMaster University in Hamilton, Ontario, demonstrated that bacteria in the gut—known as gut flora—play a role in how the body responds to stress. While the exact mechanism is unknown, certain bacteria are thought to facilitate important interactions between the gut and the brain.[7]

Gut bacteria are responsible for production of multiple vitamins including vitamin K (bone formation and blood clotting) and biotin (converts food to energy, regulates blood sugar, hair, and nail strength). They also help to regulate cholesterol metabolism and detoxify our bodies while maintaining a normal pH level in the stomach.

According to Dr. Isaac Eliaz, an integrative medical doctor, when our digestive system is not functioning properly, it can result in poor nutrient absorption/malnourishment and lead to a number of chronic problems including fatigue, IBS, constipation, bloating, acid reflux, autoimmune disorders, learning disabilities, and more.

The gut has its own nervous system that allows it to operate independently from the brain. This enteric nervous system is known among researchers as the "gut brain." It controls organs including the pancreas and gall bladder via nerve connections and is responsible for many of our feelings and emotions.

"A Gut Check for Many Ailments," a great article by Shirley S. Wang about the connections between digestion and emotions, was published in the *Wall Street Journal* in January 2012. The article mentioned the scientific research indicating how problems in the gut may cause problems in the brain, just as a mental ailment, such as anxiety, can upset the stomach.[8] What you think is going on in your head may be caused by what's happening in your gut. Besides being responsible for nutrient absorption, our digestive system acts as a major source of neurotransmitters—the chemicals that determine our emotional state. Researchers call the enteric nervous system the "gut brain" and note that about 95 percent of the neurotransmitter serotonin is produced by neurons in the gut.[9]

Besides serotonin, other neurotransmitters are directly dependent on the health of our gut, including GABA, endorphins, dopamine, epinephrine, and norepinephrine. Each of these neurotransmitters has a different effect on mood, depending on the supply of amino acid fuel available. Serotonin makes us feel positive, easy-going, confident, and enthusiastic. When its production is hindered, due to gut inflammation, we can feel worried, pessimistic, obsessive, irritable, and sleepless. Talk about food/mood connection!

The GI tract is an integral part of a system of organs responsible for our defense system against bad bacteria, viruses, toxins, and infections. There, specific gut-lymph tissues work with other gut immune cells to identify and kill any pathogens, toxins, or other health-robbing substances we may have ingested, as noted by Dr. Isaac Eliaz, who stressed the importance of a healthy digestion for a strong immune system.

The immune system is another function of our intricate and ingenious digestive system. Our internal delicate ecosystem controls the presence of harmful invaders and good bacteria that support our immunity. Good bacteria living in the gut are responsible for maintaining a healthy gut flora and preventing yeast overgrowth, parasites, and other harmful microbes. Healthy gut flora assists in digestion, manufacturing of vitamins, and assimilation of nutrients.

For us women, digestion is also very closely connected to self-confidence, sexuality, and our relationship with ourselves. I believe that the quality of our relationship with our bodies is reflected in the health of our digestion.

If you have ever experienced bloating, an IBS-type diarrhea, constipation, or gas, you know that confidence goes out of the window and the stomach can become the only center of attention. When digestion is unhealthy, it is natural to have resistance to being social, going out with friends, meeting new people, and you lack energy and the desire to be creative. These become a nightmare instead of a fun activity. Similarly, most careers require public appearances, networking, and a lot of interaction. If all of your thoughts are focused on your belly and trying to choose food that will reduce the distress, it is difficult to engage with people on a deep level. Deep connection comes from the core of our being. When our core, our center, is inflamed and in pain, deep connection is impossible.

Sexuality and digestion have a close tie, as well. Most women with whom I work on the issues of digestion and emotional eating also have experienced some degree of difficulty with achieving orgasms, have experienced low libido, and often have had irregular periods. I am not a doctor and can't tell you if there is a physiological connection between poor digestion and the reproductive system, even though my guess is there is. What I know as a woman is that feeling feminine, sexy, playful, and flirty is almost impossible when we feel bad about our own body. A distended stomach, cramps, feeling stuck down there from carrying around several days of waste, burping, and a feeling of heaviness after a meal is anything but sexy. It kills the desire for intimacy!

A healthy belly that feels light, nourished, and calm creates a much better base for intimate connection. When you can breathe fully into your belly without feeling like a balloon that is about to pop, you can connect to the lower energy centers in your body, which are responsible for helping you feel sexual, feminine, and motherly. It also makes sex a lot more enjoyable because you can be fully present in your body and with your partner instead of worrying about your stomach.

Digestion and relationship with self is another important point. As a woman, I know that women's state of digestion influences their internal dialogue. Many women engage in a self-loathing internal dialogue with their body if their stomach is expanded or bloated and painful. They think something must be wrong with them.

Self-loathing leads to more emotional eating and to worse digestion. Bad digestion and an inflamed gut lead to more ruminating about food and more negative self-talk. We've got a very negative cycle here! I am not saying that healing your gut will automatically create an immense feeling of self-love and acceptance, but it makes it easier. We will also talk about ways that you can make the process of healing stem from a place of love and compassion for your body versus turning it into a restrictive medical diet.

If you remember one thing about the importance of taking care of your digestion, remember this: your body is a vehicle that allows you to create the change in the world that you want to see and to enjoy many of life's pleasures. The state of your body is largely determined by the state of your digestion. If your digestion is assimilating nutrients, your body is building healthy cells and blood. If your digestion eliminates all the waste efficiently and in a timely way, you enjoy a clear mind and vibrant energy. When you take care of your digestion, your body enters an optimal thriving state from which you can step into your full potential, mentally, physically, and emotionally.

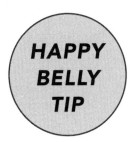

Functions of the Digestive System/Gut Brain

- Building new cells and blood
- Healthy skin, hair, and nails
- Learning abilities, ability to focus, and memory
- Bone formation
- Production of neurotransmitters (serotonin, GABA, melatonin, etc.)
- Mood, energy level, sleep

chapter 2

MY STORY

Unfortunately, I didn't start writing and researching natural ways to heal digestion because I wanted to help women suffering from bloating, constipation, and emotional eating.

My relentless research and experimentation came out of desperation. It was a strong desire, a need, to feel better.

From my early teenage years I had issues with digestion. My belly never was my close friend. We would always fight. I put more food in than necessary, and my stomach would make me feel shitty by holding on to all the crap (literally) and poisoning my body and my mood. We were not in a good relationship. I would go as far as saying it was a mutually abusive relationship.

Throughout that time, I was searching for answers to help me understand why my stomach was giving me so much trouble. I wanted to know why a simple physiological function that should happen automatically preoccupied such a big part of my brain and felt so nasty in my body, why foods that were supposed to be "good" for me irritated my gut and made me look five months pregnant;

why certain foods felt heavy as a brick while other foods sucked all the energy out of my body instead of nourishing me.

As a busy graduate school student, I had no interest in spending hours rolled into a ball on my couch, babying my tummy instead of studying, working, or having fun with my friends!

I also hated the fear of ballooning up after a dinner. There is no worse mood killer than a bloated stomach. I didn't want my social relationships to suffer because of my digestion issues.

In my effort to "fix" my gut, I embarked on a long journey filled with dietary experiments: fiber supplements, detoxes, fasting once a week, green juices, probiotics, enzymes, macrobiotic diet, lean protein diet, raw food diet, herbal teas, essential oils … Some of them were helpful; some were a waste of time and energy. Nothing seemed to resolve all the issues entirely. Some things were effective but totally not practical. At one point, I made my boyfriend carry single-serve probiotic drinks in his suitcase every time we traveled (and we traveled every weekend!).

Sometimes I felt hopeless and angry at my body for putting me through such a challenging journey, and other times I felt inspired to be learning at such a fast pace in a hands-on way.

Throughout this journey, I was hoping to, one day, find a plan that would help me and my belly feel healthy and happy. I wanted to have a list of foods to eat and not eat, recipes to make, exercises to do, herbs to take — anything and everything that would help and be effective without being ridiculous. And I wanted it presented in a clear, easy-to-follow manner.

After years of experimenting and learning about my body, my belly and I are in a much more evolved, loving relationship. I feed it well; it doesn't get bloated or constipated. I massage with warm oil, which makes my entire body feel healthy and light because food is digested quickly and easily. Thanks to my ayurvedic teachers, holistic doctors, coaches, and meditation instructors, I am now able to see a bigger picture of how my body breaks down and what it needs to get back into a balanced state. It goes beyond choosing the right diet or taking supplements, even though those are very important.

To share everything I learned along the way and to help other women (and men) who might be having digestive issues, I created this very special and dear-to-me book. I hope that it will save years of painful experimentation and research for those who are struggling with digestive unease. If it saves someone a day of feeling unpleasantly full from not going to the bathroom regularly or being bloated after a "healthy" meal or waking up puffy and groggy, I will consider my mission accomplished!

At the time of writing this book, my digestion is regular, my stomach feels flat and nourished, and I feel pretty confident about my food choices. Finally, I don't feel restricted or controlling around food. Eating is not a math problem of figuring protein, fat, and carb ratios. Instead, I feel adventurous, playful, and relaxed when it comes to meals. I look forward to cooking and eating.

Most of all, I love sharing the strategies that worked for me with my clients and friends! In the last three years, I've seen amazing transformations in women of all ages using principles that I will describe in this book. You can read some inspirational stories at www.spinachandyoga/healingstories.

Am I at the end of my healing journey? Probably not. I don't know if there is ever an end. As humans, we get quickly acclimated to a new better "normal" and then continuously look for ways to improve it. While, for someone with severe constipation, going to the bathroom once in three days is "normal," I wouldn't settle for anything other than at least once a day, preferably early in the morning and after drinking some warm water. This is my new "normal," and the only way I want to go from here is to a better state of digestion and health.

Considering our environment, the frequency of eating out, questionable sources of food, and crazy levels of stress, I don't think it is realistic to say that I will never feel bloated again. Neither will you, unfortunately. But what you and I can do is to learn habits and recipes that will help us get into balance a lot quicker. So instead of spending three days constipated, you will skip only one day at the most; instead of feeling bloated and miserable for days at a time, you can feel better within minutes or hours. It is all about adapting to the environment and doing the best with what we have, not about being perfect.

Our wounds are our best teachers. For a long time my belly felt like a painful, uncomfortable, energy-sucking wound. It took a lot of work and time to understand the physical and emotional causes that brought digestive discomfort and pain. Now I hope to share what I learned on my journey of making friends with my body and healing my digestion from constant bloating, chronic constipation, and guilt-inducing, gas-producing emotional eating.

chapter 3

INVITATION TO TAKE RESPONSIBILITY

As a society we are used to handing over responsibility for our health to doctors or alternative medicine practitioners. *They should know more about our body than we do and they get paid to keep us well. They have the knowledge of what pills we should take, what foods to eat, and how much to exercise.*

If this is what you believe, it is time to reconsider.

Nobody cares about your state of health and your energy level as much as you do. Even the kindest doctor, nutritionist, or wellness coach has limited time and not a lot of control over your health. Even if they are committed to help you, they can't force you to change your habits until you take an active stance and responsibility for how you feel living inside your body.

Nobody but you has control over many aspects of your life. While conventional doctors or alternative medicine practitioners can offer you medicine or herbs, they cannot control your thoughts or emotions. They can't watch over your eating habits either.

Your health and well-being depends on YOU. You are responsible for learning how your digestion works or doesn't work. You also have the power to improve your health and digestion if you set your mind to it. Throughout your journey, keep these guidelines in mind:

- Be willing to explore and experiment.

- Don't rush.

- Don't try to be perfect or know it all.

- Find a like-minded community in your local geographical area, or on social media, that you can use for inspiration and support.

- Pay attention to the emotional aspects of healing as much as to the physical ones.

- Be ready to let go of the old beliefs about your health, digestion, and food.

- Be forgiving and gentle on your body and mind.

- Restart and recommit to your journey as many times as needed. Changing habits is not easy. Small failures are nothing but a good lesson that will help you to move forward. Don't let the failures discourage you. Commit to doing the best you can every morning.

If you feel that you are ready to take responsibility for how you feel and help your body feel and look amazing, let's start by evaluating the state of your digestion.

chapter 4

HOW HEALTHY IS YOUR GUT?

B y now you know that vibrant health, great energy, and an overall healthy body is unachievable without a healthy digestive system. But how do you know whether your gut is healthy and doing its job?

A good way to determine your current health and the health of your gut is to ask yourself a few simple questions: *How do I feel inside my body? Is it comfortable? Light? Easy to move? Does it have a lot of energy? Is my stomach light and nourished or bloated and heavy? How do I feel when I think about food and eating?*

Dr. Pam Popper, the author of *Food Over Medicine*,[10] offers a wonderful way to determine if your digestion requires attention and healing. When your digestive system is healthy and is functioning well, you should not be aware of its work. If you are conscious or aware of the process of digestion from the moment you put food in your mouth to the time you eliminate it, there is something going on. Whether you feel the discomfort in the upper part of your digestive tract, anywhere in the stomach or intestine area, or are having trouble eliminating regularly, something is not working the way nature has intended. Dr. Popper says that digestion should be something we don't ever have to think about. Our bodies are designed to silently do the work for us upon the ingestion of food. Yet for many of us, digesting food is far from unnoticeable.

I also put together a short and simple questionnaire that will help you learn more about your body and the state of your digestive system. Pain and severe discomfort are not the only determinants of digestive problems. Most often the symptoms start in a very mild form. Many people live with chronic digestive symptoms and are used to them. However, it is not a normal state of being. A healthy digestive system should not cause any discomfort to you.

Take a pen and let's find out how your belly is doing!

UNDERSTANDING THE STATE OF YOUR DIGESTION

Digestion Questionnaire

1. How often do you go to the bathroom?

☐ less than once a day

☐ one to three times a day

☐ more than three times day

2. Do you experience any of the following? (check all that apply)

☐ burning or heat sensation in your throat or stomach

☐ bloating or flatulence

☐ fatigue after eating

☐ diarrhea

☐ fullness and a heavy feeling for extended time after meals

☐ cramps after eating

☐ abdominal pain related to food

☐ sour taste in mouth

☐ regurgitation of undigested food into mouth

☐ burning sensation from citrus on way to stomach

☐ heartburn

☐ burping

☐ difficulty passing stool

☐ bad breath

☐ bad body odor

☐ chronic or frequent fatigue or tiredness

☐ food allergies, food sensitivities, or intolerances

☐ sinus or nasal congestion

☐ chronic or frequent inflammations

☐ eczema, skin rashes, or hives

☐ chronic nasal congestion

☐ intolerance to greasy foods

☐ headaches after eating

☐ fatigue and sleepiness after eating

3. **What does your stool look like?** (yep, you have to examine the evidence before flushing it down!)

☐ looks like a banana and is "S"-shaped

☐ thin and almost thread-like

☐ hard balls

☐ soft/liquid mush

4. What is the consistency of your stool?

☐ mucus in stools

☐ similar to toothpaste

☐ poorly formed

☐ pieces of undigested food in stool

☐ blood in stool

5. How would you describe your appetite?

☐ strong and regular

☐ tend to eat when stressed

☐ variable: some days strong, some days no appetite

☐ no appetite; eat because I have to

6. How many times a day do you sit down to eat a meal?

☐ less than one time a day

☐ one to three times a day

☐ more than three times day

7. How long does it take you to finish the meal?

☐ less than 10 minutes

☐ 10–20 minutes

☐ more than 20 minutes

8. How many times a day do you eat without the phone, TV, or computer on?

☐ less than once a day

☐ one to three times a day

☐ more than three times day

9. How often do you find yourself still hungry after a meal?

☐ less than once a day

☐ one to three times a day

☐ more than three times day

10. How often do you eat because it is "time to eat" but not when you are hungry?

☐ less than once a day

☐ one to three times a day

☐ more than three times a day

11. How many times per week do you eat a meal with a larger portion size than you feel is healthy?

☐ almost never

☐ one to two times

☐ three to four times

☐ five to six times

☐ seven or more times

12. Do you have a history of:

☐ ulcers or gastritis

☐ current ulcers

☐ vaginal yeast infections

☐ antibiotic use

☐ use of nonsteroidal anti-inflammatory drugs (aspirin, Tylenol, etc.)

☐ increased sensitivity from drinking alcohol

☐ headaches or migraine headaches connected to food

DIGESTION QUESTIONNAIRE KEY

1. How often do you go to the bathroom?

A healthy person should eliminate at least once a day. Anything less is considered constipation according to integrative and holistic practitioners. While Western medicine considers two times a week "normal," it is not optimal for health. Just think about it for a moment. Whatever you eat and don't eliminate has to stay inside your body in 98-degree heat. The longer it stays there, the more likely it is to start fermenting and creating gas, bloating, and eventually toxins.

2. Do you experience any of the things on this list?

Each check mark on this list indicates that your digestion is in a less-than-optimal state. The more responses you check off, the more likely you would benefit from actively embarking on a Happy Belly program and bringing your digestion back into balance before it leads to unpleasant health consequences.

3. What does your stool look like?

A healthy stool should be well formed, brown in color, and shaped somewhat like a banana. If it is hard and dry, you are most likely constipated; soft, mushy stool may indicate indigestion, food allergy, or diarrhea. Thin and almost thread-like stool could be a sign of an inflamed, swollen gut and resulting constipation. Evacuation should not be painful or burn. It should feel satisfying and easy.

4. What is the consistency of your stool?

Stool should be well-formed. If there is blood in your stool, you should call your doctor! Pieces of undigested food in stool—unless it is skin from hard-to-digest fruits and veggies—can signify poor chewing.

5. How would you describe your appetite?

Strong and regular is a sign of good digestion. If you tend to eat when stressed or angry, you are more likely to experience indigestion. Variable appetite could point to IBS or indigestion. Lack of appetite could signify high toxicity, poor or sluggish digestion, or constipation. When there is no appetite, don't eat! Let your digestion rest and use the energy for detoxifying and healing.

6. How many times a day do you sit down to eat a meal?

Ideally, you should be eating every meal sitting down, not in the car, standing up, or walking. Your digestion requires a lot of circulation, so if your body is forced to be doing other things besides chewing and digesting, your digestion will suffer.

7. How long does it take you to finish the meal?

If you chew your food well and don't rush to finish your meal first, it should take 20–30 minutes. If it takes longer, it's fine. If it takes you only ten minutes to eat, you are more likely to feel unsatisfied after the meal, have cravings, and suffer from indigestion. If you don't chew your food, your stomach has a lot more work to do. As a result, your energy levels, after a meal, may go down.

8. How many times a day do you eat without the phone, TV, or computer on?

We are constantly busy and rarely find time to put our phones down or eat away from the computer. Unfortunately, it has a very negative effect on our digestion. We eat a lot more when we are not fully present, feel less satisfied, and are more likely to hinder digestion.

9. How often do you find yourself still hungry after a meal?

It is important to learn how to eat balanced, nourishing meals that leave you feeling satisfied and energized.

10. How often do you eat because it is "time to eat" but not when you are hungry?

If you eat when you're not hungry, you are going against your body's signals; you are not respecting your body's voice. It is best to eat when you are hungry and your digestion is ready to take in food.

11. How many times per week do you eat a meal with larger portion sizes than you feel are healthy?

Overeating is one of the worst things we can do for our digestion. The more frequently you overeat, the more likely you are to experience digestive unease.

12. Do you have a history of

Ulcers or gastritis, diagnosed food allergy or food sensitivities, or intolerances? Intolerance to greasy foods may signify a weakened digestive system that requires particular care. Vaginal yeast infection, antibiotic use, chronic or frequent fatigue or tiredness, sinus or nasal congestion—these can be due to an unhealthy gut flora or yeast overgrowth. Use of nonsteroidal anti-inflammatory drugs, alcohol, and processed foods contribute to bacterial overgrowth. Bad breath and body odor, eczema, skin rashes, hives, and chronic or frequent inflammations may be a sign of acidity. Alcohol sensitivity can be due to an overloaded liver. Headaches or migraines connected to certain foods, fatigue and sleepiness after eating may be due to a food sensitivity or allergy.

Besides doing the questionnaire, examining your tongue is another great way to assess the state of your digestion.

chapter 5

WHAT IS YOUR TONGUE TELLING YOU?

When I was a little girl, my parents, who both were doctors, always asked me to show my tongue if I complained of not feeling well. I don't know if you remember, but several decades ago doctors in Western hospitals also examined patients' tongues as one of the first diagnostic steps.

More than 10 years later, I finally started to learn exactly what my parents and doctors were looking for. The tongue is a detailed health map. Our tongues change colors/shades, shape, and surface texture, providing a current health status update. Tongue analysis is an ancient health assessment technique that is still used in Chinese medicine and by ayurveda practitioners.

Much as in reflexology, different parts of the tongue correspond to different organs. As a mirror of the body's digestive system, the tongue can reflect the toxicity level in the gut, show potential food sensitivities or a weak digestive fire, point to malabsorption of nutrients, and reveal the health of other organs in the body.

Trained ayurvedic practitioners will be able to provide a complete health analysis by examining a patient's tongue. Dr. Vasant Lad,[11] the founder of the Ayurvedic Institute in New Mexico and one of my favorite ayurvedic teachers, encourages everyone to learn the basic tongue diagnosis principles as they can serve as a useful health analysis tool. Our tongues contain a wealth of information, and learning how to interpret the looks of our tongues can be very helpful in understanding our bodies on a deeper level. It is a great way to build a closer mind/body relationship. Any trusting healthy relationship has to be based on mutual understanding.

A daily look at the tongue helps us to become more aware of the effects of food on our body. The tongue doesn't lie. It provides the feedback about last night's dinner with full honesty first thing in the morning. This is your free daily health report.

The beauty of a tongue diagnosis is that its basics can be learned and applied by anyone to monitor their own health. While it might take years to learn the intricacies of tongue diagnosis, there are some general guidelines that anyone can use to evaluate general health and digestion.

Dr. Lad advises you to look at your tongue in the morning before brushing your teeth. He also strongly encourages the use of a tongue scraper on a daily basis. Why walk around with a ton of toxins if you can just scrape them off?

Scraping the tongue first thing in the morning removes overnight build-up of bacteria and toxins. Rather than brushing the tongue, which will only push bacteria and toxins into the tongue, scrape your tongue with a tongue scraper or spoon. You can use a metal or a copper one. To scrape your tongue, extend it out and place the scraper as far back on the tongue as comfortable.

Using one long stroke, gently pull the scraper forward so that it removes the unwanted coating on the tongue. Rinse the scraper and begin again if necessary. I usually do it five to six times.

There are a few factors that are worth noting when you look at your tongue: shape, shadings, markings, wetness, texture, and coating. A healthy tongue should look like a kitten's tongue or a young baby's tongue: symmetrical and evenly pink. It should not tremble. It should have a thin, transparent coating. All the taste buds should be flat, orderly, and free from bumps, lines, cracks, and patches. It should not have foam, hair, fur, be too dry, or too wet, or have a foul odor or taste.

If you want to learn the intricacies of tongue diagnosis, I highly recommend getting the book *Ayurvedic Tongue Diagnosis* by Walter Santree Kacera.[12]

As a beginning tongue explorer, there are a few things you should pay attention to:

Tongue coating. Excessive coating usually means sluggish digestion and toxins in the colon. Depending on the food that you eat, coating will change from day to day. If you have a late night heavy dinner of pasta and wine, your tongue is more likely to be swollen and have a thicker coating. This is the way your body is trying to tell you that the digestive system might be overburdened. Knowing that your colon is full of material that doesn't belong there, that spreads toxins into your blood, makes you sluggish, your skin dull, and your head foggy might be exactly what you were waiting for in order to change your diet. If you wake up with a heavily coated tongue, take a break from heavy, oily, and processed foods and choose foods that are easiest to digest until the coating clears up.

Teeth imprints. Teeth imprints around the contour of the tongue can mean malabsorption of nutrients, inflammation, or too much salt in the diet. If your tongue has teeth imprints, your digestive system is not very happy. Most likely it is overloaded and weak. To stimulate digestion in a natural healthy way, add fresh ginger tea, avoid iced drinks, and start paying attention to food combining, which we will discuss later in the book.

Trembling tongue. This is a sign of anxiety or fear. We live in such a high-stress society that anxiety can crawl over you without you even being aware of it. It might even be your permanent state and you are so used to it that you can't tell the difference. Time to take a break from caffeine, have some chamomile tea, and nourish your nervous system with warm and easy-to-digest light soups.

The changes on the tongue will show the effects of changes in your diet. You will be able to watch the changes on your tongue as you begin healing your digestion.

Now that you have an idea about the state of your digestion and you know how important a healthy gut is to your health and happiness, let's talk about a few things that might be causing digestive unease and discuss strategies that will help you improve your digestion.

part 2

WHAT CREATES AN UNHEALTHY GUT?

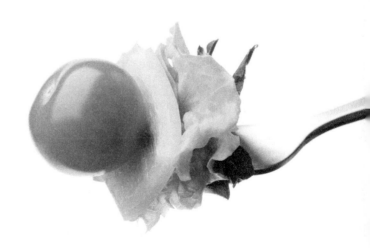

chapter 6

HOW DID IT GET SO BAD?

L et's look at a few things that could potentially trigger digestive unease. They include bloating, constipation, IBS, diarrhea, and acid reflux. Years of research, interviewing experts on nutrition and digestive health, multiple lectures, workshops, and endless experimentation have helped me pinpoint a few things that can irritate the digestive system and create digestive unease.

There are many factors that influence the health of our digestive system. It is important to remember that we are complex beings in which all the systems and organs are interconnected and interdependent. We are also highly dependent on our environment. Our internal microcosm is constantly interacting with the external macrocosm. This highly sophisticated interaction of various organs within our body, external environment, and emotions and thoughts, creates a huge list of factors that could potentially hinder or improve digestion.

The digestive system consists of multiple organs that have to work in sync to break down the food, assimilate the nutrients, and expel the waste. This intricate, beautifully designed system has been perfected by evolution over millions of years. As a highly effective team, all the relevant organs—including mouth, esophagus, gall-bladder, stomach, liver, pancreas, intestines, and veins providing the necessary blood flow—influence the efficiency of your digestion. Each team member has to do its job well and on time for the outcome to be successful. If even one of the team members is weak and unable to perform its function, or is eliminated by accident or surgery, the result might be problematic.

Besides internal factors, such as the health of each organ involved in digestion, there are also lots of external factors to consider. The quality and the amount of food, the time of eating, climate, age, stress, medications, and physical activity all have an impact on digestion.

We tend to forget that we are whole living beings. We grow up in a culture where things and people are highly specialized and compartmentalized. When it comes to our body, we think of various organs fulfilling their functions. We perceive them as functioning independently of each other. The stomach digests food; the liver breaks down fat, protein, and alcohol; the brain thinks; the heart pumps the blood. All of this should happen automatically and effectively.

In reality, all the organs and internal systems are very much interconnected and interdependent. They make up a highly intel-ligent human body. When you take medicine for your head, it will affect your liver and digestion. Whatever you put into your stomach will affect your brain and nervous system. There is no division or separation within the body. The mental division of various organs and systems is created by modern medicine where every doctor is highly specialized and knows only about his particular part of the body. While a heart doctor, a GI specialist, and an endocrinologist might function as separate doctors, within your body, those organs are not separated. You are one, and you are whole. Accepting this knowledge means that you accept the effect of your environment on your digestion, the intricate connection between your gut and emotions, and the powerful effect of your thoughts and stress level on your health.

It may be hard to fully accept the nature of existing as an integral being and to apply it to daily living. Many of us believe that the digestive system is separate from the rest of our body. In a way, we equate our stomach with a trashcan. We throw in some good stuff, some bad stuff, some supplements, and pills and then don't care about what happens after the mouth is closed. We hope that something good will turn out. We believe that nature will do its work. We forget that whatever went into the stomach will soon affect our mood, energy, hormones, and emotions.

When your digestion is bothering you, it might be tempting to reach for the quickest and easiest solution that will help to relieve pain, bloating, constipation, or heartburn. However, dealing with symptoms is only half the battle. It is very important to figure out which one of the variables that influences digestion is not in balance.

Before jumping to fix things, it is important to figure out where the weakest link is for you. It might be an internal factor such as a habit around food that you got from childhood, or it can be an external factor such as a bad relationship with your boss. Quite often there is a strong link between the functioning of the internal organs such as intestines and liver and external factors such as stress levels, the amount and quality of food, or presence of chemicals in the environment. This makes the importance of a holistic approach to healing very important. The best results require tackling the problem from multiple angles.

In the next several chapters, we will talk about various internal and external factors that may have a negative effect on the functioning of the digestive system. Read through each one and then see which one is more relevant to your situation. Most of this book is about helping your digestive system heal, but understanding what causes pain and discomfort is also really important.

Over the last several generations, many of the external factors that influence digestion have been dramatically changed. What we eat has changed. How we eat has changed and how often we eat has changed. As a result, our digestive system is forced to adapt to a completely new way of functioning, which it sometimes has a difficult time doing.

I will go over a few factors that have changed dramatically, and you, in turn, should try to imagine what and how often you would eat if you lived as a hunter/gatherer or an early agrarian, thousands of years ago. Just let your mind wander off into the ancient times. See through the eyes of that ancient man or woman the challenges of getting food, the celebration of food when it was abundant, and the starvation times when food would only be given to the weak and the children. Close your eyes and let your imagination take you on a ride.

chapter 7

....

ACTING AGAINST EVOLUTION

Our diet has changed dramatically in volume and substance from what our ancestors used to eat.

"Most of us no longer have to eat whatever we can get compared to our starving ancestors. On the contrary, we may eat whatever we want—but what we seem most often to choose is an ever-narrowing range of foods that are mostly sweet, or high in fat content, or low in dietary fibers. Our digestive system, which evolved to deal with scarcity and variety, is now called upon to handle abundance and nutritional uniformity," writes Deepak Chopra in his book *Perfect Digestion*.[13]

We went from a high-fiber, whole-foods diet to a diet of overly processed grains and fats with lots of sugar and salt. We also went from eating ceremonially and appreciating every morsel of food to rushed, mindless eating in front of the TV while watching terrifying news reports.

There are more chemicals in our food, and a good portion of food is fully or partially processed. We also have food available 24/7 and don't have to expend as much energy to hunt for it. We don't go through the regular starvation periods to which our ancestors were accustomed, and the quantity of food we consume is way more than our great-great-grandfathers could have ever dreamed of. Many traditional cultures and some modern-day health practitioners recommend reducing the amount of food on a seasonal basis to give our digestive system a much-needed rest.

According to the US Department of Agriculture food consumption report of 2012, the average American eats literally a ton of food each year, or about 2,700 calories each day—and an alarming proportion of that is sugar and other sweeteners.[14] That includes 29 pounds of french fries, 23 pounds of pizza, 24 pounds of ice cream, 53 gallons of soda, 24 pounds of artificial sweeteners,[15] 2,736 grams of salt, and 90,700 milligrams of caffeine per year. Do we really think we can maintain a healthy digestion with this much toxic food? With a total of 632 pounds of dairy products per year, 85 pounds of fat and oils, and 134.1 pounds of wheat flour in an average standard American diet (SAD),[16] our digestion is up for some serious, never-before-experienced challenges.

We also combine foods in ways that our ancestors could not have dreamed about. Can you imagine a primal man searching the grounds for the ingredients to make a burrito or a pizza pie? I doubt our ancestors had a chance to enjoy multiple-course menus. Most of the food was most likely very simple and consisted of just two to three ingredients, if that! And this is what our digestive system is used to.

There is a lot to be grateful for since we are living in times of abundance compared to the ancient times. We have a lot more time on our hands to be creative, to develop spiritually, to travel, and to work on projects that ignite our passion rather than fight for our day-to-day survival. However, our gluttonous nature that was created in times of scarcity and starvation often gets our digestive system in trouble in these times when there is too much abundance.

Our relationship with, and appreciation of, food has shifted significantly over the last several centuries too. Constant availability of food and its historically low prices make us less appreciative of every meal. That, in turn, transforms us into mindless eaters. Try imagining growing your own vegetables, weeding them, watering them from the nearest pond, and protecting them from the bugs. I bet you would appreciate those veggies a lot more if you had to do that much work to obtain them.

When I was a kid, my parents bought a house in the country so we could spend time outside and eat homegrown produce. I am so deeply grateful to them for doing that. They had no experience in farming or in taking care of animals, but they took a leap and my sisters and I grew up running around in nature. We also tried our hand taking care of our own veggies, chickens, ducks, turkeys, rabbits, pigs, cows, and a big garden.

We witnessed baby cows being born, drank fresh unpasteurized milk from a cow that we tried to milk ourselves, went to pick berries in the spring, and ate fresh greens directly from the garden. Now that I think about it, the whole lifestyle that our parents created for us was as close to a natural, seasonal way of living as it could get. Fruits were in season at the end of the summer, and we rarely had them at other times. This made the imported mandarins at New Year's smell like heaven. We would eat one per day, making sure that they lasted, and save the peels to make tea because they smelled so good! Now most of us are used to having any fruit at any season. There is rarely a deep sense of appreciation for getting something in the supermarket because you haven't waited for months to get it.

While I grew up eating meat, chicken, eggs, and dairy in the years at the country house, this meat always came from our own animals. It was always served as a special occasion and as a center dish. It was not "chicken with some veggies"; it was "veggies with some chicken." If an animal was killed, every single part had to be used because the animal's life was deeply appreciated.

Another factor that has changed quite a bit is how we eat. We usually do it in rush, without chewing and while playing on the phone or checking Facebook. We basically went from eating in a ceremonious way with a family or a tribe to eating with a computer and a phone. Mindless eating, which we will discuss in detail further in the book, can lead to overeating and problems with digestion.

Our digestion is very adaptable. Throughout history, various geographical tribes had very different diets. Some had extremely high-fiber, plant-based diets with only occasional animal protein present, and other cultures ate predominantly high-fat, meat-based diets. Until the introduction of modern processed foods, elevated stress levels, and an overabundance of cheap food, most of those tribes were very healthy.

As an example of the extreme, Eskimos ate 99 percent raw animal products and lived free of degenerative disease before white men introduced them to cooking cauldrons, breads, and refined sugar.[17] According to accounts of world travelers and explorers, Eskimos were considered the happiest of all races. Their first reported case of dental decay came 50 years after cauldrons, breads, and refined sugar were introduced.

At the other extreme are cultures that lived on predominantly high-fiber plants, roots, seeds, nuts, and fruit. Until the introduction of modern-day foods and ways of eating, these cultures were also healthy and strong.

Whole foods have become a thing of the past unless all meals are cooked from scratch. Even some health-conscious brands add chemicals, flavor enhancers, soy, sugar, and wheat gluten to almost every item. Along with processed foods filled with flavorings and various taste enhancers, our taste buds have become somewhat desensitized. Desensitized taste buds require stronger tastes. Natural, simple food may seem bland and tasteless to the taste buds that are used to strong, often chemically induced flavors. The good thing is that taste buds renew very quickly. After four to five days of simple foods, fruit becomes heavenly sweet, and plain steamed veggies taste amazing. Our bodies regain their ability to classify foods into good and not so good for the body. We have an inborn ability to tell whether the food is beneficial for our bodies or if it is detrimental. We just forgot how to trust this innate ability because we have grown accustomed to having someone else tell us what to do. Remembering might take time and trust, but it is definitely possible!

chapter 8

BAD EATING HABITS

S elf-destructive behaviors lead to destruction.

It's a simple, logical way that things always play out. If we were to analyze our lives, we would see that we do a lot of self-destructive things on a regular basis.

They include eating hard-to-digest, almost nonfood-like substances our ancestors never could imagine eating; breathing bad air; not moving; drinking strange-colored drinks and alcohol; stressing out; not sleeping enough; getting angry; taking drugs; and smoking. Then we are surprised when we get sick, tired, and can't poop.

Fortunately, the opposite is also true: when we engage in self-healing activities, our body heals.

Through societal laws, family traditions, parents' eating patterns, and our own childhood and adulthood experiences, we form habits around eating that can hinder or support digestion.

Many of our habits surrounding food are unconscious and changing them is not always easy, even when we know a change is good for us. Often our digestive system can deal with one or even a couple of harmful eating habits for quite a long time. The stronger our digestion, the more it can handle. Layering harmful habits one on top of the other creates more difficulties and disease over time.

For example, overeating is bad, but with enough rest before the next meal, our body can handle it once in a while. Chewing food poorly is also undesirable for the digestion, but our digestion can work through it.

Layering overeating and not chewing is a lot harder on the gut. It leaves the stomach with an uncomfortable amount of food that is swallowed in large chunks. It will take a lot of energy and time to digest and will most likely leave a person feeling very sluggish.

Let's layer it a bit further. Imagine a large meal, late at night, that is poorly combined with hard-to-digest ingredients, accompanied with a large, iced, carbonated drink, followed with a heavy dessert, eaten in front of the TV while you are feeling upset and angry about work not going so well. This is setting the stage for indigestion, heartburn, a heavy unpleasant feeling in the stomach, and sluggish energy the next morning.

Bad eating habits can hinder digestion even if you eat all organic, pure, healthy food. They can be as much of a reason for indigestion as the food itself. This is why we will discuss a few eating habits that can have a negative effect on the process of digestion, and at the end of the chapter, you will be able to evaluate your own habits around food.

How one eats is just as important as what one eats. Specifically, the quality of digestion is related to what is going on in the mind, in the body, in our environment, and in our emotions. When one is not focused in the mind while eating—thinking about work or other things—the energy of digestion is diverted away from the activity of digestion. If one is emotionally charged while eating, the sympathetic nervous-system functioning dominates: blood supply is shunted to the peripheral muscles and away from the stomach.

Digestive juices stop flowing, and the peristalsis of elimination stops. When the body-mind is at rest, the parasympathetic nervous system dominates and digestion and elimination proceed normally.

When reading about eating habits, try not to engage in self-blame, shame, or any sort of mental self-mutilation. Your habits are often the result of your social surroundings, lack of knowledge, and patterns that you inherited from your parents. It is not your fault that you have them. You can, however, create new habits that will help your digestion and health in general. New healthy habits will, over time, replace the old ones. So, one step at a time, let's take a look at some habits that hinder digestion.

HARD-TO-DIGEST FOOD COMBINATIONS: DISEASE OF OVERABUNDANCE

Many of the food combinations we consume on a daily basis, multiple times a day, would be impossible in nature.

For a long time I have been noticing that not everything that I eat makes me feel equally well. The more I pay attention to my stomach before and after food, the more information my body provides. While I am still learning to decipher my body's feedback, one finding keeps emerging more often than others: THE SIMPLER THE DISH, THE LESS ENERGY IT REQUIRES TO DIGEST — which means there is more energy left to do other things such as write, think, teach, do yoga, and just enjoy life.

Simplicity is key to many effective strategies. Digestion is no different.

You may eat a vegan diet and still get gas or feel bloated. Food sensitivities aside, improper food combinations can be one of the major reasons behind belly troubles. Those who voluntarily eliminate certain food groups from their diet (for example, dairy, gluten, flesh, eggs) are less likely to confuse digestion with improper food combinations. Those courageous, strong-willed people have fewer food groups to combine in their meal. They have less choice. It makes their diet simpler and therefore more digestion friendly.

However, you don't necessarily have to eliminate entire food groups to keep your belly happy. Also, going gluten-free or vegan doesn't necessarily mean that you don't have to look into food combinations, especially if you want to increase your energy levels.

If you think about it, our ancestors were not very likely to combine multiple food groups in one meal. If they found berries, they ate berries. If they were lucky to hunt something down, they had a feast of meat or game. I can't imagine ancient people cooking side dishes, dressings, and desserts in a cave kitchen. Our ancestors ate mostly simple monomeals, consisting of one to three ingredients at a time.

Each food that is taken into our body requires different enzymes to digest. Different foods also require different amounts of time to be digested. Fats and carbs all need their own particles that help to break them down. The pancreas works really hard to make all those enzymes available. A meal consisting of multiple ingredients from different food groups will require the most enzymes and the most time.

If the pancreas is overloaded or weak, there won't be enough enzymes to break down the food. This is one of the reasons that people who start taking enzymes as a supplement usually feel they are able to digest their food better. However, taking enzymes is controversial, and while it is supported by some nutritionists and doctors practicing functional medicine, others would say that it can hinder the natural enzyme production within the body. An ayurvedic practitioner, John Douillard, in his article "The Hidden Danger of Digestive Enzymes,"[18] talks about a dependency that may develop in the body if people take enzymes with every meal. Over time, people may require larger and larger doses of digestive enzymes with every meal. Instead of relying on pills, Douillard recommends strengthening natural enzyme production and digestion. Avoiding difficult-to-digest food combinations will help to strengthen digestion over time. Drinking a big glass of water with lime juice 15 to 20 minutes before each meal will help hydrate the stomach, encouraging it to produce more hydrochloric acid and increasing the flow of bile and pancreatic enzymes.

Food combining can be applied to any diet to reduce post-meal digestive unease, improve elimination, resolve skin issues, and increase energy levels. One of the ways to make sure that you get a positive net gain of energy from food is to eat nutrient-dense, easily digestible foods. Another way is to make sure that those nutrients can be easily absorbed into your body by keeping food combinations simple.

Later in this book, in the section on healing digestion, we will talk about simple food combination rules you can include in your daily eating. Before we get there, it might be helpful to take a look at some of the worst food combinations that are very common in most people's diets.

TEN COMMON FOOD COMBINATIONS
THAT WREAK HAVOC ON YOUR HEALTH

I chose 10 food combinations that are considered hard-to-digest by followers of ayurveda—the Indian science of life and health—natural hygienists, and physiologists. Basically, people who care about their body and digestion would never think of eating these foods together on a regular basis if they knew what happens in their digestive system.

Some of the immediate consequences of bad food combinations are digestive unease, gas, bloating, stomachache, nausea, fatigue, and constipation. While short-term effects can clear up within a day or two, long-term poor food combining can lead to more severe problems such as bad breath, dry skin, rashes, chronic inflammation, poor sleep, low energy, and chronic digestion issues. Most people feel a surge of energy and naturally lose weight once they start following several simple food-combining rules, which we will discuss later in the book.

Here are some popular items on the average American menu that present a big challenge to our body and can wreak havoc on your health.

1. **Fruit after a meal.** Natural hygienists have known for a long time that fruit doesn't combine well with other foods. Modern-day holistic GI experts, such as Donna Gates, the author of *The Body Ecology Diet*, agree. The reason is that fruit contains simple sugars that require very little time to be digested. Thus, they will not stay for a long time in the stomach. Proteins are digested mainly in the stomach and hydrochloric acid is used to break them down. Carbs and fats are digested further down in the digestive tract. So if you eat fruit after a meal that contains

protein, the fruit sugar will stay for too long in the stomach until the protein is broken down, creating a bubbly, bloated stomach.

2. **Lasagna or Grilled Cheese Sandwich.** Animal protein-starch combos inhibit salivary digestion of starch. Protein and starches are digested in different areas of the stomach and need different enzymes and different levels of acidity to be digested. When eaten together, your body is forced to digest protein first in the stomach and starches later in the intestines. Our body can't separate starches and protein into separate batches to be broken down, so the process becomes a lot more taxing in terms of energy requirement. According to Dr. Herbert Shelton, the champion of original, natural hygiene concepts, undigested starchy food undergoes fermentation and decomposition and over time leads to poisonous end products.

3. **Cheese and meat omelet with toast.** In general, protein/protein combinations are not recommended. One single concentrated protein per meal is easier to digest and won't require as much energy. Go for a veggie omelet instead. Adding carbs to the protein meal will require a longer time and more energy for digestion.

4. **Tomato and cheese pasta sauce.** Tomatoes are considered acidic and should not be mixed with starchy carbs such as pasta. Food combining theory recommends avoiding mixing carbohydrates with acids. Adding dairy to this already difficult combo turns it into a recipe for digestive problems and after-meal fatigue, since your body will require a ton of energy to digest this meal. Have pasta with pesto and grilled veggies instead! If you are

feeling extra healthy, go for brown rice, mung beans, black beans, or quinoa pasta.

5. **Cereal or oatmeal with milk and orange juice.** Acids in orange juice or any acid fruits destroy the enzyme that is responsible for digesting starches in cereal. Also, acidic fruits or juices can curdle milk and turn it into a heavy, mucus-forming substance. To keep your breakfast healthy, try having fruit or orange juice 30 minutes before the oatmeal.

6. **Beans and cheese.** Dairy protein and beans are a common combo in Mexican cuisine. Eaten with a hearty serving of sour cream and hot sauce, it is almost guaranteed to lead to feeling sluggish afterward, and gas and bloating. It is not the beans on their own that cause it, but the combination as a whole. Try skipping cheese and tomatoes if you have weak digestion or are working on detoxifying your body. Add some zucchini and mixed greens and stick to one protein.

7. **Melon and prosciutto.** Melons should be eaten alone or left alone. The same rule goes for all high-sugar fruits. In general, it is preferable to eat fruits separately from proteins or starches, especially if you are looking for a quick energy boost.

8. **Bananas and milk.** Ayurveda lists this combination as one of the heaviest and most toxin-forming. It is said to create heaviness in the body and slow down the mind. If you are a fan of milk-based banana smoothies, make sure the banana is very ripe and add cardamom and nutmeg to stimulate digestion. Go for nut or seed milk instead.

9. Yogurt with fruit. Ayurveda and food-combining theory don't advise mixing any sour fruits with dairy as it can diminish digestive fire, change the intestinal flora, produce toxins, and cause sinus congestion, cold, cough, and allergies. Ayurveda suggests avoiding congestive and digestive fire-dampening foods such as cold yogurt mixed with fruits. However, if you can't resist the temptation of a yogurt parfait, there are ways to make it more digestion friendly. First of all, go for a room temperature, natural, unflavored yogurt. Second, mix a little bit of honey, cinnamon, and raisins instead of sour berries.

10. Fruit-flavored ice cream. Similarly to yogurt, this dairy and fruit combo is also extremely mucus producing, heavy, and hard to digest. The ice-cold temperature will make the digestion process even more energy-consuming. Having ice cream after a meal will create fatigue and heaviness in the stomach, and could lead to a runny nose, congestion, and sluggishness. Keep ice cream seasonal; in the summer, have it as a separate meal during the daytime, and go for either fruit sorbet, home-made banana ice cream (www.spinachandyoga.com/recipes), or get good-quality chocolate or vanilla gelato.

Of course, everyone has a different body and will experience various levels of sensitivity to bad food combinations. Many people attribute digestive problems and food sensitivities to particular foods while in reality it is the combination of foods that is to blame. Also, many of us are so used to digestive discomfort that we don't know what it feels like not to experience it. Everything becomes clear in comparison. If you follow simple food-combining rules for two weeks and let your digestive system rest, your digestion will be a lot more efficient, cravings will subside, there will be more energy, and a flatter belly.

For proper food combining rules, refer to the photo section in the middle of the book.

MINDLESS AND EMOTIONAL EATING

Mindless, emotional eating is often triggered by stress, negative emotions, discontent with the present state or situation and by the lack of connection to the body.

In a mindless state, when our mind is anywhere but in the body, we can engage in abusive eating behaviors such as overeating, eating without chewing, eating when not hungry, or eating as an escape from unpleasant feelings.

When we are connected to the body and committed to treating it well, it is difficult to eat to the point of a distended belly because it is uncomfortable and not pleasant. It is also difficult to eat "bad" food when you are chewing each bite with full awareness and attention. Overly processed food turns into a disgusting mush in a few seconds of chewing, and the body quickly registers how unpleasant it is. However, when eaten quickly, we can often overindulge in processed food and actually find it tasty.

When we are kids, being mindful comes naturally. We are connected to the breath and our body much more and have less social pressure to follow rules around eating. That is, until our parents start "teaching" us "proper" eating habits. Kids usually trust their feeling of being hungry or not hungry. They intuitively know when it is best to let the body rest from food and when they need some extra. Throughout the years of "bringing up" we get more attuned to behaving according to social norms and less attuned to our body. Our mind becomes focused a lot more on the outside world, not on the internal state. We start eating "by the clock," clean our plates no matter the portions, rely on research and experts' advice about what should go on our plates, and pay attention to our laptops, TVs, or phones more than our belly during meals.

It doesn't take long before we become almost fully disconnected from our bodies and dependent on outside sources to tell us what to eat, how much to eat, when to eat, how we feel, and what we need to feel better. Unless the body is screaming and yelling with pain to get attention, we grow deaf to its internal voice.

Mindless eating is the opposite of slow, mindful savoring. It is the opposite of enjoyment and deep satisfaction that the food should create. Mindless eating usually creates discomfort in the stomach and an unpleasant mental state filled with guilt and self-hatred. If *mindful* eating is slow, expansive, meditative, and nourishing, *mindless* eating is rushed, constrictive, and anything but pleasant.

When eating becomes mindless, overeating becomes routine, and binge eating can become a habit. Overeating and binge eating lead to bloating, poor digestion, internal distrust and lack of confidence in ourselves, and eventual weight gain. Your stomach will be uncomfortable and bloated whether you overeat on carrots or cookies. Overeating by itself is very traumatizing to digestion. Eating vegetables mindlessly might be less harmful because there are fewer toxins in them than in chips, but neither will make your belly happy.

Mindless eating habits often start innocently by eating on the go or eating while multitasking. Eating in front of the computer or with a phone in your hands is the same as having dinner with your partner when all he does is play on his phone. You feel lonely and ignored.

That's how our body feels during mindless meals when our minds are anywhere but in the body and with the food.

By not paying attention to the body, we lose access to one of the best teachers and guides. Our bodies have a lot of the answers that we keep looking for in books, workshops, lectures—anywhere but inside. We would save a lot of time and money if we paid as much attention to what our body tells us during meals as we do to Facebook and e-mail.

It might be one of the most difficult habits to change, but unless you commit to eating mindfully without distractions, you will always come back to the same issues with your body. Often we are tempted to play on our phone or be distracted in any other way, so long as we are not alone with ourselves because it is unpleasant, uncomfortable, and often scary. When we take time to slow down, serve the food on a plate, eat at a table, and be fully present with our meal, a lot of emotions can come up and we will have to deal with them. In search of making things better or getting away from an unpleasant emotion, we look for the quickest way of increasing our happiness levels. Eating is usually the easiest answer.

Mindful eating requires attention to the food itself, to its flavors, aromas, colors, presentation, and to the way your body responds to the food. Throughout the entire meal the connection between your body and you should never be lost. This allows you to be very sensitive to your body's feedback, which prompts satisfaction at the end of meal.

If you are distracted while eating, not paying attention to your body and food, the only way you'll know when to stop eating is if you follow strict portion control or if there is no more food left on the plate or in the cupboard. External factors dictate your decisions more than your wise body.

You know that you eat mindlessly if you find yourself uncomfortably full after a meal, when you feel empty even after a big portion of food, when you are craving for "something" even after a balanced meal, and when you feel guilty for overeating to the point of discomfort.

EATING IN A RUSH

Imagine this picture: a woman standing in the kitchen after a stressful day at work, with her husband, kids, and a dog all asking for dinner. She feels pressured, tense, and sucked into a whirlpool of things to do. She is holding her breath while hurriedly preparing dinner, replying to her husband's questions about her day, trying to ask her kids about their homework, and with the dog brushing against her legs asking for treats. She finally gets dinner on the table, gets drinks for everyone, cleans up the counter, and by the time she sits down, the rest of her family is half-way through the meal. She is so hungry by now that she just inhales her food in 10 minutes. Without breathing, chewing, or checking in with her body, she pushes the food inside to get the grounding she needs after running around all day.

Or how about this one: a student who eats while she is late for school, chewing while walking, and paying attention mostly to the road not the food or her body.

There are lots of other scenarios: eating in between meetings while checking e-mails, eating while in the car, during business meetings, while walking, or in the subway.

Eating in a rush and an uncomfortable, unhappy belly go hand in hand.

We forget that our day is limited to 24 hours and fill it up with meetings, to-do lists, and pointless time wasters just to find that there is no time left to cook or eat. Look at your days from your past week. How often did you feel rushed? How many meals did you eat on the go, in a car, or standing up?

We live in a busy, tightly scheduled, always-in-a-rush society at least five days out of seven. Meetings, deadlines, family responsibilities, errands, and social life stretch the capacities of our calendars and our physical and mental ones, as well.

Whether it's working nonstop to finish a project, running to a meeting, or rushing to a yoga class, it seems as if we're almost always short on time. If only the day had an extra few hours, we say. I think even if it had another 10 hours, we would still be in a rush because we have forgotten how not to be. With so much to do, and so little time, we don't have time to take care of our basic needs such as sleep, proper nutrition, and fresh air.

Our bodies, functioning on 90 minutes less sleep a day than even our great-grandparents had, are running fast toward damaged cardiovascular disease, weak immune system, indigestion, chronic constipation, irritability, and depression.

Often when the day gets superbusy we end up eating without taking a break from all the "important" tasks on hand. Sometimes we feel the need to scroll through e-mails while shoving in a deli sandwich or to drink soup while running to the next meeting. We are not eating mindfully while multitasking. Eating this way, we get the calories but not the real nourishment that our body and soul need. The lack of nourishment can show up as cravings for sweet foods, lack of enthusiasm and motivation, and a general feeling of dissatisfaction.

Carefully cooked and slowly eaten family meals are luxuries that not many choose to prioritize. Our bodies pay for it heavily with disturbed digestion, constant cravings for more, and an urge to overeat when we finally do sit down at the table.

Slowing down is not easy when everything around us is moving at such a fast pace. However, the slow food movement is gaining more and more fans all over the world. There are slow food parties, restaurants, conferences, and support groups. We can also start to slow down at home. Just implementing small things, such as not eating while moving or standing, cooking as many meals as possible, and not using our phones (which means no checking Facebook!) while eating can already make a huge difference.

It's hard to find enough time between work, family, and all the errands to sit down and eat a meal, but it is important for healthy digestion. It is also important for emotional health and a trusting mind-body connection. Taking time to sit down and mindfully chew your food will make the body-nourishing process a lot more efficient. You will feel full faster and longer, enjoy your food more, and your digestive system will function better. Our digestion starts in the mouth when food is broken down by the enzymes in your saliva, so the longer you can chew, the less work your stomach has to do. Starting today, promise yourself at least one sit-down meal a day!

Try to pay attention to your digestion after slow and rushed meals. If you notice a difference, then commit to make more time for nourishing your body.

GRAZING ALL DAY

The concept of snacks and frequent meals is often recommended for weight loss, maintaining blood-sugar levels, and bodybuilding. It works for some people, especially those with hypoglycemia and those who actually can keep their meals small. However, most people use the advice to eat five to six times a day as a permission to snack in between their good-sized breakfast, lunch, and dinner. As a result, they often eat way more than the body needs and overload their digestion. They also put their body in a regimen where it doesn't burn stored fat efficiently for energy. Frequent supply of food makes the body reliant on the incoming sugar for energy. Whatever is stored in the fat cells stays there.

As one of my favorite ayurvedic teachers, Dr. Vasant Lad says: the effect of eating before the previous meal is digested is similar to constantly adding beans to boiling chili. The soup never gets fully cooked. Some beans will be overcooked and mushy, and some will stay raw and hard.

In our stomach, gastric emptying doesn't occur before the food is digested enough to proceed to the next stage. If you keep adding more food that needs to be digested, than gastric emptying is delayed in order to process new food. The food that is already digested starts brewing and fermenting, creating gas.

The length of time that you should wait before eating something else depends on the meal. Different food takes a different amount of time to be digested (see the *Food Transit Times* table in the photo section). Fruit digests quickly while meat is on the other end of scale and digests much longer. You can eat another meal within 30 to 60 minutes after having fruit. Mixed protein and starch meals will require more time to digest, so you should wait longer after this meal before eating anything else. Eating multiple complex meals every day keeps our digestion always busy and leaves less energy to do the necessary housekeeping and detoxifying. Overloaded digestion is a quick road to an unhappy belly.

Traditionally, most societies ate two to three meals per day with no snacks besides fruit. Eating six meals per day is a mostly American experiment that fits the interests of food manufacturers whose desire is to make people eat as much as possible. The more we eat, the more money they make. So of course, there is a huge booming industry of snack foods and nutrition bars, as if we will drop dead if we don't eat for four hours.

As Dr. John Douillard, the founder of LifeSpa and an ayurvedic authority, correctly notes, with blood sugar levels artificially propped up from constant feeding, the ability to make energy last is replaced with fragile energy, constant hunger, mood instability, and extreme cravings if a meal or snack is missed. He also points out that having erratic eating habits, such as "grazing all day," keeps our digestive fire always on and soon the incessant digestive process begins to irritate the intestinal wall.

Also, eating six healthy meals per day is a labor-intensive process. Planning all the meals, preparing them, and properly chewing might as well take a huge portion of the day! A lot of my clients always complain that they find themselves thinking about food nonstop. Carefully planning every meal takes up most of their thinking and creative ability. There is so much more we can do with our time if we are not constantly focusing on food or digesting food.

I personally find that eating five times per day makes me think about food all the time, and I end up spending my day either cooking, cleaning up after eating, chewing, or resting after food. There is very little time left to be productive and focus on the important things.

If your blood sugar is normal, eating three to four times a day helps to keep digestion functioning optimally. Many older people will even notice that they feel better on two meals per day. It is a personal preference and should not be forced, however.

Many people find relief from digestive problems just by giving their body enough time to process foods. Usually, energy levels will be more stable throughout the day if you are not dependent on the next snack to keep your blood sugar levels stable.

After giving my body a long enough break after heavy or hard-to-digest meals, I get a surge of energy and my stomach feels light. Eating meals every two hours—unless it's simple fruit or plain vegetables—puts me in a permanent food coma where all the energy goes to digesting food and none is left for my brain to function. Grazing all day also makes my stomach bloated and uncomfortable, which never happens if I allow four to five hours between meals.

If you are used to eating throughout the day, start paying attention to your reasoning behind it and its effects.

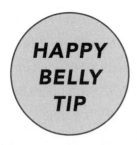

Do an experiment for a week when you eat three good-sized, balanced meals and one snack. Pay attention to how you feel toward the end of the week. The first few days might be challenging, since your body will need to adapt to a new way of eating, but once it does, you should feel a surge of energy, lighter stomach, and less brain fog.

COLD OR ICED WATER DURING MEALS

Americans love ice cubes! I have never seen any other nation so greedy for ice in drinks! Ice gets most of the space in the glass no matter what is being drunk. A social norm in all US and Canadian restaurants is to serve ice-cold water during meals. If you have ever been to Europe and Asia, you know that most restaurants and families never add ice to their drinks; even if you ask for ice, all you get is a couple of ice cubes.

Why so much love for ice cubes? It might be an American "more is always better" mentality. I never had ice in my drinks until I came to the United States. In Russia we had tea with food and after food. I grew up with my parents guarding me from ice-cold drinks as if they were deadly. My mom even warmed up ice cream for my sisters and me over the stove, turning it into lukewarm cream. It still tasted pretty good but was definitely not icy anymore!

According to an Eastern perspective, cold water slows down digestion and is likely to leave you with a heavy feeling in your stomach (even after a light meal). Ayurveda agrees.

Think of what happens if you put a cube of ice to the skin. It becomes white because all the blood flows away and blood vessels constrict. Our digestion requires a huge amount of blood flow to digest food well. This is one of the reasons that it is difficult to stay sharp mentally after a huge, heavy meal: all the blood moves into the belly away from the brain. When we pour a tall glass of iced water into the stomach along with food, it is hard to imagine blood circulation being optimal. It will require more energy for the body to warm up the water and to digest food. As a result, there might be more fatigue and brain fog after a meal.

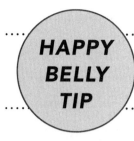

HAPPY BELLY TIP

Take small sips of warm water or herbal tea with meals.

You can drink a glass of room temperature water 20 minutes before each meal to rehydrate and awaken your entire digestive system.

ANALYZE YOUR HABITS

Now that you know that habits can have a powerful effect on the way we feel and the way our gut functions, let's take an active step toward healing.

Take a look at your eating habits. Are you eating in a rush, stressed, at the computer, not chewing your food, and past the fullness cues? Then that's where you need to start. Changing what you eat will be a lot easier if you eat slowly and mindfully while paying attention to your body cues. The desire to eat a dozen cookies will just drop away by itself.

There is no need to blame gluten, dairy, enzyme deficiency, and other things if your eating habits are not supporting a healthy digestion to begin with.

I did this for several years. I kept looking for a trigger food to blame, searching for a magic pill to make me better. For a period of time it would help, but as soon as I was stressed and stuffed myself with "healthy almonds and dark chocolate," my bloating would come back. No gluten, no dairy, no eggs, no legumes, nothing besides lean protein, veggies, and fruits and I would still suffer.

This was me until I got honest with myself and asked my body what it was that I was doing so wrong. What was it that kept ruining all my efforts to have healthy, efficient digestion and a trusting, mind-body relationship? My body whispered that I needed to slow down when I eat, to focus on chewing, not on my e-mail, relax after meals for a few minutes, and breathe all along.

Your body can give you your prescription too, if you ask and listen. Lissa Rankin wrote an entire book about it, *Mind Over Medicine*,[19] which I highly recommend. It might take time to hear your body's voice but be willing to wait because nobody knows you better than you do.

Write out the habits that you have around food:

- What habits do you have around food and eating?
- What habits are serving your body?
- What habits are hindering digestion?
- What habits would you like to give up? (Start with one.)
- Any particular habits you would like to adopt?

Make a commitment. Write a promise to yourself:

I promise to _____

Now go back to the questions and write them out before reading any further!

chapter 9

STRESS AND DIGESTION

S tress is another huge factor in digestive health. Most of us are perpetually stressed. Living in a fight or flight mode doesn't allow our body to digest food properly. Digestion is optimal in a "rest and digest" state, which is the opposite of the "fight-or-flight" mode. If you are eating a mostly whole foods diet and give your body enough time to digest it and still experience on-and-off digestive unease, chances are good that your body is stressed. According to Kenneth Koch, MD, professor of medicine and medical director of the Digestive Health Center at Wake Forest University Baptist Medical Center in Winston-Salem, North Carolina, our digestion is closely connected with the central nervous system. When our nervous system is under stress, our digestion can shut down.

Marc David, the founder of the Institute for the Psychology of Eating, says that the key to understanding the profound link between digestion and stress is the central nervous system (CNS). According to Marc David, the portion of the CNS that exerts the greatest influence on gastrointestinal function is called the autonomic nervous system (ANS). This aspect of the nervous system is responsible for getting your stomach churning, the enzymatic secretions in the digestive process flowing, and keeping the dynamic process of nutrient absorption into the bloodstream on the move. The ANS also tells your body when not to be in digesting mode, such as when there's no food in your belly or when you're in fight-or-flight response. The same part of our brain that turns on stress turns off digestion. The part of the brain that turns on the relaxation response turns on full, healthy digestive power.

HAPPY BELLY TIP The more stressed, tired, sleep-deprived, or anxious you are, the more foods will aggravate your digestive balance.

Our autonomic nervous system has two subdivisions: the sympathetic and parasympathetic branches. The sympathetic branch activates the stress response and suppresses digestive activity. The parasympathetic branch relaxes the body and activates digestion.

A lot of people lose their appetites when they're stressed out. But oftentimes, they end up eating anyway because they don't want to skip a meal. (Unfortunately, many of us are convinced that skipping meals is a sin and that our body will stop functioning if we don't feed it every two hours.) The body is a lot smarter than that.

During stressful situations, our nervous system is wired to shut down blood flow to the digestive organs, decrease secretions needed for digestion, and cause different contractions of our digestive muscles. Forcing down food at this time would not be a good idea!

Think of an important business lunch or a job interview over dinner. If you are nervous and your body is in fight-or-flight mode, digestion will not be a priority.

Trust your body's intuition and eat only when you're truly physically hungry. Eating while stressed, scared, and angry won't help. If you can, wait until you're less stressed and then celebrate with a beautiful meal. Some might fear that skipping meals is unhealthy, others that they will get bellyaches, dizziness, and fatigue, or worse, that they will drop dead from missing one meal! In reality, staying without food for more than four hours is not that scary, especially if you are busy.

I am not trying to talk you into fasting when you are hungry, though. Quite the opposite: if you are hungry, and it is a true physical hunger, eat! On the other hand, when we are under a lot of pressure and stress, the hunger can be less-than-normal. It happens because our body is trying to keep all the energy for the to-do list and has very little energy left to digest food. Eating at this time simply would be not efficient.

If you are in a perpetual high-stress mode, your goal should be to nourish your body at the times when the stress levels are a little lower. It means having your biggest meal when you are less tired and not as busy. During the peak times, keep your food liquid and easy to digest. Liquid-based foods provide an easier-to-access source of nutrition. Keep it light and nourishing.

We rarely can control the circumstances or problems that come up at work, but we do have control over how we perceive things and how we nourish our body during stressful times. As a general rule the more stressed you are, the gentler diet you should follow. Your biggest meal should be when you are less tired and not as busy. Help your body to deal with stress by reducing energy-draining heavy foods.

Here are a few easy-to-digest foods that you can eat during stressful days

- herbed vegetable and/or chicken soup or clear fish soup with vegetables (no dairy and low sodium). Try one of the soups in the color insert.

- red lentil soup (green or brown lentil is a lot harder to digest)

- nondairy vegetable curry

- berries

- stewed fruit

- fresh juicy fruits

- spiced almond milk blended with dates and spices

- porridge with vegetables or quinoa with vegetables

- steamed veggies with a piece of wild salmon

- room temperature smoothie without dairy or too many nuts

And here are some foods to avoid because they are considered hard to digest

- dry nuts and crackers

- sandwiches

- burritos

- quesadillas

- pizzas

- pastries

- heavy meat-based dishes

- anything with cheese

- anything cold, dry, or not freshly made

This is one of the areas where you need to do an honest experiment and stick with the option that works better. It might mean that you choose to have a good, filling breakfast, a light lunch at work, and a bigger but easy-to-digest and simple dinner when you are in a relaxed environment at home. A bigger dinner is not ideal since our digestion is naturally weaker during the evening, but you have to do the best with the circumstances you are facing. Having a big lunch during a stressful day in front of the computer and no break afterward is cruel to your digestive system and to your productivity.

chapter 10

FOOD SENSITIVITIES

Food sensitivity is an interesting and very important topic. While I have first-hand experience with food sensitivities, before I talk about my experience, I would like to share a perspective regarding food sensitivities from a triple-certified functional nutritionist, Dana James, the founder of Food Coach NYC, a close friend, and an amazing specialist who clarified this topic for me when I was puzzled by reactions to certain supposedly "healthy" foods. Her explanation follows.

Our body is an innately intelligent vehicle that has trillions of cells working towards restoring balance and harmony. Every nano-second of the day it is absorbing and assimilating nutrients; it is expelling waste, creating micro-flora for our gastrointestinal (GI) tract, defending us from pathogenic bacteria and fungi, creating hormones, enzymes and neurotransmitters to communicate to our cells and detoxifying endogenous and exogenous chemicals. Our body has its own internal pharmacy. All we need to do is give it the nutrients it needs to be able to function optimally and take out those things that are causing any imbalances.

Food sensitivities and intolerances are significant contributors to inflammation and imbalance in the body. A food sensitivity is a delayed hyper-immune response to a particular food. The reaction can manifest anywhere from 20 minutes to 48 hours later. It is this delay that makes it challenging to identify what the problematic food is.

It is thought that approximately 40 percent of the American population has an undiagnosed food sensitivity. Gluten is the most common allergen, with dairy being second. An intolerance, such as lactose intolerance, is a digestive enzyme deficiency. About 20 percent of the population has such a deficiency.

Both of these are distinctly different to an allergy, which produces an acute and severe response, such as hives and anaphylactic shock. Approximately 2 percent of the population has a food allergy, with the most common offenders being peanuts and shellfish. Food allergies are Ig-E mediated by the immune system. They are not a major cause of distress in the body because their reaction is so violent when ingested that the person vigilantly avoids the food.

A food sensitivity develops when an undigested protein molecule erroneously enters the blood stream. Only protein that has been fully broken down to individual amino acids, dipeptides or tripeptides should cross into the blood stream. The body correctly perceives this food to be foreign and mounts an immune response to destroy and remove the offending molecule, much like it would a bacteria or a virus. This releases pro-inflammatory cytokines to neutralize the food, which can lead to a cascade of physical and neurological symptoms. The symptoms can range from almost non-detectable to debilitating. They include IBS, IBD, abdominal bloating, diarrhea, constipation, migraines, depression, anxiety, ADD, violence, weight gain, insulin resistance, food addictions, cravings, autoimmune disorders, PMS, tongue swelling, joint pain and water retention.

How your body responds to a food sensitivity depends on your current biochemistry and this response may change over time. It may start as a digestive reaction but lead to neurological symptoms and insulin resistance. This means it might initially present with IBS and then lead to anxiety and weight gain. As you reverse the food sensitivity, the symptoms start to dissipate and may only manifest as inflamed gums if you eat the offending food. From what I've witnessed in my practice, dairy tends to produce IBS, diarrhea, and sinus congestion. Gluten tends to produce all other symptoms. Food addictions, cravings, neurological disorders and joint pain tend to exclusively be the realm of gluten.

Other foods, such as brewer's yeast, almonds, and lemons, can become allergens, not just gluten and dairy. However, I rarely see a person without a gluten or dairy sensitivity. Perhaps 2% of the clients I test have a sensitivity to foods that don't include either gluten or dairy. The reason for this is that gluten and the protein molecules in dairy are large molecules. The larger the molecule, the more likely it will not be broken down to its constituent components and therefore the more likely it is to cause inflammation in the GI tract and allow these molecules into the bloodstream. Once the lining of GI tract has been compromised by these abrasive molecules, it opens the door for other foods to slip into the bloodstream. This is called leaky gut or intestinal permeability.

To understand the interaction of food and leaky gut, think of the lining of the GI tract as a bouncer at an elite club. He is there to let well-dressed and attractive people in while keeping the riffraff out. If, however, some burly men charge at the bouncer and beat him up, then the burly men could slip into the exclusive club. If it was just a few of the burly men, the "coolness" of the club would unlikely be compromised, but if the burley men called 100 of their other friends to run amuck then the club would lose its prestige and become a little ugly, much like the state of your immune system once the GI lining is damaged.

The longer the lining of the GI tract is damaged the more foods the body adversely reacts to and the more inflammation is triggered setting the stage for autoimmune conditions, including celiac disease. Celiac disease should not be confused with a gluten sensitivity. A gluten sensitivity will always precede celiac disease. Celiac disease is an autoimmune condition whereby the villi of the small intestine have atrophied due to excessive exposure to wheat and its gluten molecule, gliadin. Testing for celiac disease to see if you have a gluten sensitivity is like testing for diabetes to see if you have elevated fasting glucose levels. The damage is done well before you'll show a positive result.

In my practice, testing for food sensitivities has been one of the most powerful interventions to reverse a whole spectrum of chronic conditions. I use a test that looks at the cytokine (white blood cells) reaction to specific foods. It identifies the severity of the reaction and by the number of sensitivities you can determine how permeable the gut is. The more foods that show up, the more leaky the gut is. If someone presents with a large number of foods, I work on healing the GI tract first and taking out four of the most allergenic foods. Often fixing the GI lining will reverse some of the minor sensitivities without the need to exclude them.

When I initially tested myself back in 2007, I was shocked by the sheer number of foods I was sensitive to. Surely this had to be wrong? I wasn't presenting with any digestive distress (the most common symptom) but I wasn't sleeping well, lacked the vibrancy I normally imbued and felt if I didn't run in the morning, I'd be a little blue. I put this down to moving countries, writing my dissertation, going through a divorce and starting my nutrition practice without any USA-based contacts. I was in denial. So much so that I didn't even think I was stressed because I was "handling" it.

But my body was smarter than my brain and it was telling me to pay attention to it. I ignored it.

By the time I re-ran the food sensitivity test three years later the permeability of my gut had increased exponentially, my cellular inflammation was rampant, and I'd gone from being mildly sensitive to gluten to being moderately sensitive. I'd also developed a dairy sensitivity. I was bloated, puffy, and had morning sinus congestion thanks to the very small amount of milk in my daily coffee. I was living a life that was both gluten and dairy light, so the transition to gluten and dairy-free shouldn't have been much of a jump, but I met it with extraordinary resistance.

I realized I had to listen to the advice I gave my own clients: "If you don't take gluten out of your diet, you'll become a celiac." With that wake-up call, I took out both gluten and dairy and a couple of other random food sensitivities. I healed the gut permeability and improved my adrenal function. The sinus congestion went away in a week, the bloating dissipated, I lost those lingering last three pounds and I was no longer a slave to carbohydrate cravings. I had balance back in my life.

How do we end up with food sensitivities? Stress is the greatest influencer. When we are stressed, the body goes into a sympathetic mode turning on adrenaline and cortisol to cope with the stressors. This sends blood pumping around our body, heightens our awareness, and slows down our digestive function. This physiological response harks back to our cave-man days when we were either fighting or fleeing a wild animal. We needed to be on high alert and ready to run towards or away from the stressor. Digestion was not the priority. That happened when we were calm and safe back at our camp.

This physiological preference has not changed over the last 500 generations, even though the stressors we encounter are different. Being in a constant state of stress, even if it is low grade, will interfere with the body's ability to produce stomach acid and digestive enzymes that are crucial for breaking down food to its constituent components so that it can be absorbed and assimilated in the body. When the food is not broken down fully, the larger molecules start to wear away at the GI lining, causing permeability and allowing these undigested food molecules to enter the blood stream, triggering inflammation and establishing a food sensitivity (or two or 100). At the same time, the lower levels of stomach acid kill off fewer bacteria, viruses, and fungi. These microbes produce toxins, which also increase the permeability of the gut lining.

There is a widely accepted belief that the more stressed you are, the more stomach acid you produce. Physiologically, that's not how it works. You actually produce less because digestion is not the priority. Acid reflux happens not because of excess acid but because stress strips the body of magnesium and magnesium is required to hold the sphincter between the esophagus and stomach tight to prevent acid going back into the esophagus. When this sphincter is loose, acid goes up into the esophagus, creating acid reflux. The solution is to tighten the sphincter; it's not necessary take acid blocking medication. Acid blocking medication not only inhibits stomach acid, but it also decreases the release of digestive enzymes, since stomach acid sends a signal to the pancreas to release the digestive enzymes.

This, in combination with the increase in pathogenic toxic-relaxing microbes, creates the perfect storm for GI permeability, food sensitivities, and a whole host of inflammation.

Constant exposure to a particular food also increases your likelihood of a sensitivity, particularly if there is already GI permeability. If you are eating cereal for breakfast, followed by a sandwich for lunch, pretzels as an afternoon snack and pasta for dinner, then you've got wheat, wheat and wheat at every single meal. Or perhaps your diet is a little more sophisticated than this. You have granola for breakfast, salad sandwich on spelt bread for lunch, high-fiber crackers with avocado as an afternoon snack and fish and vegetables for dinner with a bite of bread (you know, you can't resist). This diet may be more nutrient dense, but it still has gluten in it at every meal. Gluten includes oats, wheat, barley, and rye.

Frequent consumption of alcohol also increases the likelihood of a food sensitivity. When alcohol is metabolized, it creates a highly volatile toxin called acetaldehyde and if this molecule is not neutralized quickly, it can damage the lining of the GI tract, thereby allowing food into the bloodstream.

The pervasive use of antibiotics in our medical system as well as food supply creates a breeding ground for pathogenic microbes that produce toxic by-products which compromise the GI lining.

The good news is that we weren't born with food sensitivities and therefore we can reverse them. We do this by identifying what they are, restoring GI integrity, and improving the microbial balance in the GI tract.

. . . .

I am sure you learned a lot from Dana's words! She is a gem!

Now, I would like to share my perspective and experience with food sensitivities.

As Dana mentioned, food sensitivities are caused by the "leaky gut." When the inner ecology of the gut is damaged, the cells of the intestine become inflamed. We end up absorbing very little from the food that we eat.

Donna Gates, the founder of BodyEcology and a pioneer in the digestive health field, notes that our microflora effects the health of the cells of the intestine. With bad gut flora, intestines lose their ability to do work. This means that food might sit stagnant in the small intestine, where it ferments and putrefies. The large intestine may lose motility, or the ability to move. Most importantly, the wall of the intestines becomes irritated and leaky.

Leaky gut syndrome can make foods that are supposed to be "good for us" irritating, triggering a set of unpleasant symptoms. This brings us back to the notion that I introduced in the beginning of the book: *We are not what we eat; we are what we digest and assimilate and eliminate.*

If your body is sensitive to broccoli, you will feel the negative effects of it more than the positive. Knowing this takes the importance of keeping advice personalized to a new level. What works for someone else is not guaranteed to work for your body.

One of the main aspects of food sensitivity is that we often crave foods that we are sensitive to. Our body goes through a similar withdrawal as it would with alcohol and drugs. If there are foods that you continuously crave, you most likely have a sensitivity to the food.

It happened to me with almonds. I was craving almonds almost every day. Being an ayurvedic foodie, I would soak, peel, and eat them as a snack. The only thing was that if I had them on an empty stomach, I felt tired within a few hours, as if I had been hit with a brick. Four or five hours later, the fatigue would dissipate. I never knew what this reaction was until I was tested. Now I can have almonds occasionally but definitely not as a daily snack.

In the next section, I will share some more insights about gluten and dairy, two main trigger foods when it comes to food sensitivities.

GLUTEN

Gluten-free is all the rage now. If you have recently been to a health food store you must have seen gluten-free bread, cookies, granola, and other foods. Are you wondering what this is all about? Why is a grain suddenly considered an enemy?

Gluten is a protein with sticky properties found in grains such as wheat, rye, and barley. This glue-like property makes gluten useful to the food industry, which uses it as a binder, filler, shaper, bulking agent, texturizer, and stabilizer in its products.

You would think that gluten should be found only in bread and baked goods. In reality, gluten is added to a huge variety of products from sauces to cosmetics. Nevertheless, the main gluten source is still bread. Wheat today is completely different from the wheat that our ancestors ate and even from what other countries eat now. "Wheat in the US has been hybridized to increase the yields and it has much more gluten protein in it," says Dr. Frank Lipman, the founder and director of the Eleven Eleven Wellness Center in New York City and an internationally recognized expert in the fields of integrative and functional medicine. "It's also much higher in sugars than you would realize," he says. "Eating two slices of whole wheat bread is the same as two tablespoons of sugar." The high sugar content is also what makes bread so darn hard to quit. This is just one of the reasons Dr. Lipman calls gluten "the devil." Along with its addictive sugar content, gluten is also highly inflammatory. The slicing and dicing of the gluten molecule has made the molecule larger and more robust. While this may be great for the bread, it's deleterious to our digestive system. It makes it abrasive and less likely to be fully digested, triggering inflammation of the GI tract, GI permeability, and a gluten-sensitivity.

If you have ongoing digestive issues, it is possible that you may have a gluten sensitivity. Gluten-containing foods can interfere with digestion and can contribute to immune reactions, inflammatory conditions, autoimmune disorders, neurological and behavioral illness, skin diseases, osteoporosis, chronic fatigue, and a host of other degenerative conditions.

One of the reasons that we are so sensitive to gluten is because gluten is everywhere. It is almost impossible to escape gluten in America. Dr. Lipman created a list of the most likely offenders: all-purpose flour, white flour, wheat flour, bran, cracker meal, durum flour, wheat germ. Unless labels specifically read "gluten-free," gluten is in most breads, buns, rolls, biscuits, muffins, crackers, cereals containing wheat, wheat germ, oats, barley, rye, bran, graham flour, malt, kasha, bulgur, spelt, melba toast, matzo, bread crumbs, pastry, pizza dough, pasta, rusks, dumplings, zwieback, pretzel, prepared mixes for waffles and pancakes, cakes, cookies, doughnuts, ice cream cones, pies, prepared cake and cookie mixes, bread pudding, bread stuffing or filling—anything that is breaded. Gluten also winds up in gravy and cream sauces thickened with flour, soy sauce, hydrolyzed vegetable protein, brewer's yeast (unless prepared with a sugar molasses base), yeast extract, malted drinks, beer, ale, gin, and whiskey.

Besides gluten being very difficult to digest on its own, we rarely eat it separately. We usually mix it up with other hard-to-digest, often processed foods. When was the last time you had plain wheat bread on its own with no eggs added, no butter, cream cheese, or some sort of animal protein? Being hard to digest on its own, it becomes incredibly difficult to digest mixed with other foods.

If you are stressed or tired, your digestion is tired also; in this situation, it is best to avoid gluten. If the body is expending less energy to deal with this hard-to-digest protein, it has more energy for other processes, including self-healing and detoxifying. Moreover, the liver, digestive, and immune systems are given time to rest and recover, which is why taking gluten out is so important in the process of returning people to health.

DAIRY

Milk was once considered the perfect food in many traditions, and was recommended for children, the sick, and those looking for enlightenment. Ayurvedic and ancient yoga scriptures include milk as a staple in a pure, energy-giving diet. Milk was said to nourish all body tissues, to calm the mind, and improve sleep.

Nowadays, many modern-day nutritionists and integrative-medicine doctors blame dairy for a surge in digestive disorders, obesity, internal inflammation, autoimmune disorders, acne, and hormone imbalances.

On one hand we hear proponents of dairy proclaiming that without dairy it is difficult to maintain healthy bones, and on the other hand we get promises of a better digestion and glowing skin if we go dairy-free. Some say that adults don't have the necessary enzymes to digest dairy, while others proclaim milk to be a wholesome, protein-rich food.

It is a never-ending argument that is supported by long-standing tradition, and the dairy industry, from one side, and functional medicine and the detox industry from another. I personally believe that it is impossible to give a one-size-fits-all answer about dairy. Everybody's digestive system functions differently, and we come from different backgrounds and cultures. The sources of dairy have to be considered, and the way dairy is included in the diet is important.

In general, processed, hormone- and antibiotic-filled factory-farmed dairy is not an option for consumption. If the question is about this type of dairy, the answer should be a clear no. There are more negative effects of this mucus-forming processed substance than there are positive ones. Aged, heavy cheeses should also be a rare occurrence in a healthy diet if you are not ready to give them up completely.

When combined with other heavy or cold foods, dairy becomes even harder to digest and can slow down the digestive process. Sandwiches with cheese, bread, processed meats, and mayo are extremely clogging even for the strongest digestive system. If you were to compare digesting these heavy foods to a workout, it would probably be the same as running a marathon. You wouldn't make your legs run a marathon every day, would you? So don't force your digestive system to work overtime digesting nutrient-deficient, energy-sucking food.

If you do choose to keep a little bit of dairy in your diet, make sure you are not sensitive to it by paying really close attention to your body and digestion. Keep portions small, combine young mild cheeses such as ricotta with vegetables and heating spices such as black pepper, and enjoy them during daylight hours when digestion is the strongest. Avoid combining dairy with fruit such as yogurt parfait or smoothies.

··

chapter 11

CAFFEINE

M any people drink coffee to stimulate elimination. Sorry, but this secret had to be revealed! While in the short-term coffee can help, long-term, it creates constipation.

In chronic constipation, coffee acts by overstimulating the gastro-colic reflex. Once overstimulated, the reflex loses its normal ability to be initiated by a morning glass of water, and the individual becomes dependent upon coffee to go to the bathroom.

Modern science supports the theory about coffee and constipation connection. The National Digestive Diseases Information Clearinghouse,[20] part of the National Institutes of Health, reports that caffeine can have a negative effect on digestion and lead to or exacerbate constipation. Caffeine can cause dehydration, and people experiencing constipation may experience worsened symptoms if they drink caffeinated drinks, such as coffee.

Coffee, in part because of the caffeine it contains, can generate an increase in stomach acid production. Greater amounts of stomach acid are linked to increased intestinal activity. Because IBS primarily manifests as a disorder of cramping and gastrointestinal over-reactivity, the increase in stomach acid as a result of drinking coffee can produce a marked worsening of IBS symptoms.

To explore the issue further, I found some interesting data in research papers on caffeine and GI function.[21] Coffee produces a laxative effect in susceptible people through stimulation of rectosigmoid motor activity as soon as four minutes after drinking. Even modest doses of coffee can have this effect, whether or not the body is ready to dispose of the feces, resulting in loose stools. Studies show that decaffeinated coffee has a similar stimulant effect on the GI tract, proving that the laxative effect is not only due to caffeine. Caffeinated coffee stimulates activity of the musculature of the colon and colonic motility, more so than water. Decaffeinated coffee also increases motility, although less so than caffeinated coffee.

HAPPY BELLY TIP Try Teeccino, dandelion, almond milk with carob powder, light green tea, or Matcha tea.

Dr. Samuel Hahnemann, the founder of homeopathy, also notes in his research on coffee[22] that coffee can make us less conscious of our body's natural urges to eat when hungry, to rest when tired, or to drink when thirsty. Basically, it deafens us to our internal voice to some degree.

Another very important detrimental effect of coffee, as Dr. Hahnemann notes, is that nutrient absorption can suffer because of coffee consumption. Here is a quote from Dr. Hahnemann's paper on coffee:

Our intestines, excited by coffee (in its primary action), to more rapid peristaltic movements, force their contents but half digested more quickly toward the anus, and the gourmand imagines he has discovered a splendid digestive agent. But the liquid chyme which serves to nourish the body can in this short time neither be properly altered (digested) in the stomach, nor sufficiently taken up by the absorbents in the intestinal canal; hence the mass passes through the unnaturally active bowels, without parting with more than the half of its nutritious particles for the supply of the body, and arrives at the excretory orifice still in a half-liquid state. Of a truth a most excellent digestive agent, far surpassing nature![23]

Green tea, which is a favorite of many who quit coffee, can have a stimulating effect on digestion, as well. I'm not telling you to give up caffeine altogether; I am encouraging you to experiment with reducing the amount you consume and just allowing for a possibility of life without coffee at some point.

If you drink coffee to go to the bathroom, please consider that every time you drink coffee on an empty stomach, it irritates the mucus lining of the intestines. It is not a healthy way to stimulate elimination. If you are interested in improving elimination without caffeine, try warm water with lime or lemon in the morning and sit in a squatting position for five minutes after. It will help to create downward flowing energy and stimulate elimination. We will talk in detail about regularity further in the book. If you can't imagine your life without coffee, have it after water and try to avoid having it on an empty stomach.

chapter 12

OVERABUNDANCE OF SUGAR

B y various approximations, each American consumes anywhere between 100 to 160 pounds of sugar per year—compared to only 6.3 pounds in 1822! This is a lot of sugar! Pimples, imbalanced gut flora, weight gain, hormone problems, energy ups and downs, and sugar blues are unavoidable with such high consumption.

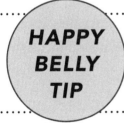

HAPPY BELLY TIP

In overabundance, sugar acts as a toxic substance that wreaks havoc on your gut health.

Sugar and its inexpensive substitutes, such as high fructose corn syrup (HFCS), are found in virtually all processed foods. We eat so much sugar and HFCS that they are the single largest source of calories for Americans. It's loaded into soft drinks, fruit juices, sports drinks, and hidden in most processed foods.

Besides weight gain, sugar creates a chronic inflammation, which has far-reaching consequences, including gut health. Sugar can spur growth of unhealthy bacteria and fool our natural body's hunger/ satiation control system. As a result, we end up addicted to sugar, always craving more. Its highly acidic effect in the body gets in the way of healing. Bad bacteria such as candida that sugar feeds can lead to bloating, fermentation, and IBS symptoms.

All these scary facts don't mean that you should never have your favorite cookie or a piece of chocolate any more. Let's be realistic. If you want to help your body heal, you would be better off replacing sugar with berries and other fruit, adding stevia instead of Splenda, and baking with date sugar or coconut crystals. Whole and less processed wins over highly processed. Fruit wins over baked goods. Raw chocolate wins over Snickers bars.

Our taste buds take just a few days to become more sensitive and to appreciate the natural sweetness of fruit versus highly processed cake. Give them a chance, and you will enjoy better health and a lot less bloating!

For wonderful, filling, and healthy dessert recipes, check out the special recipe page at www.spinachandyoga.com/recipes. You can also download a list of Happy Belly–approved sugar substitutes at www.spinachandyoga.com/resources.

....

chapter 13

MEDICINES THAT ARE HURTING YOUR GUT

A lot of over-the-counter and prescription medicines list digestive symptoms such as heartburn, constipation, nausea, or diarrhea as possible side effects. With millions of people on a daily dose of one or more medicines, it is no wonder many people make peace with experiencing digestive symptoms while taking their prescriptions.

Some of the main healthy gut enemies are antibiotics and acid blockers.

ANTIBIOTICS

Antibiotics were a life-saving invention that lengthened our lifespans and probably saved many of us multiple times per lifetime, but they also have serious negative effects on our gut flora if used too often and for a prolonged time. When antibiotics get into our system, both good and bad bacteria suffer. Healthy bacteria in the gut are crucial for a strong immune system and a healthy, well-functioning digestion.

While most doctors believe that our body restores its own balance after a course of antibiotics, more and more research proves that even a single course of a strong antibiotic can permanently alter human intestinal flora. Some bacteria might have a hard time coming back to life.

The destruction of healthy gut flora can make the mucosal lining more susceptible to leakage.[24] A lack of healthy gut bacteria is associated with allergies, IBS, and general autoimmune reactions.

Though antibiotics may be necessary in certain situations, it's important to weigh the benefits of using them with the potential risks that may come from the permanent alteration of the gut flora. If antibiotics must be used (and there are certainly situations where this is the case), special care should be taken to not only restore gut flora using probiotic foods and supplements, but to eat a diet that supports healthy gut microbiota with plenty of fermentable fibers from starch and the removal of food toxins.

Considering that most dairy and meats have traces of antibiotics, it is possible that our healthy bacteria is constantly under attack and needs periodic help of probiotics to stay healthy. This is another reason to choose organic animal products from the farmers who do not use antibiotics.

ACID BLOCKERS

Drug companies make more than $7 billion a year selling acid-suppressing medications. Every little deli and supermarket carries over-the-counter antacid medication. People pop them like candy, thinking that they are helping their body. In reality, acid-blockers promote bacterial overgrowth, weaken resistance to infection, reduce absorption of essential nutrients, and increase the likelihood of developing IBS, and other digestive disorders. The pharmaceutical companies have always been aware of these risks.

When acid-stopping drugs were first introduced, it was recommended that they not be taken for more than six weeks. Almost no one follows this precaution, and it is quite common for people to be on antacid medications for years.

Antacid medications are overused because in our society pills and quick fixes are praised and changes in lifestyle are often considered a last resort and way too challenging. For this reason, it is a lot easier to get a prescription for pills than dietary and lifestyle guidelines from the doctor. Anyone who comes in complaining of heartburn or GERD is most likely to receive a piece of paper for the pharmacy, not the farmer's market.

There are four main negative consequences of acid-stopping drugs: increased bacterial overgrowth, impaired nutrient absorption, decreased resistance to infection, increased risk of cancer and other diseases. This doesn't mean that you should stop taking all your medicines, but do consider changing your diet and lifestyle to make the medicines less needed.

part 3

HAPPY BELLY
JOURNEY

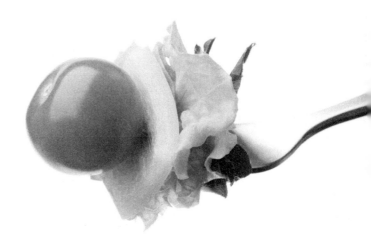

chapter 14

MAKE IT REAL

Knowledge without action won't improve your health.

It is nice to learn about your body, to read, take workshops, and talk with your friends. However, knowing something and doing something is very different. We all know that we should eat lots of veggies, exercise regularly, and be polite, but not everyone does it. Why? Because it takes a lot of clarity on priorities, consistent effort, mindfulness, and daily practice.

The same is true for healing digestion. Knowledge is not enough. Daily action is required if you want to see a positive change. I know you can do it, and I want to help you find the easiest, least stressful way to get to where you want to be.

These actions will guarantee your success in getting back to innate digestive health:

- Be clear on how you would like to feel and why.

- Identify obstacles that you might face and outline ways you can overcome them.

- Be mindful and attentive to your body's signals.

- Commit to daily practices (food log, movement, creating and re-evaluating your weekly goals).

- Participate in a supportive group
  (family or Happy Belly community online at
  www.facebook.com/spinachandyoga).

- Relax and/or meditate daily.

- Be patient and willing to forgive yourself and start over every single time that you go back to old habits.

Think of this journey as your way to recommit to your body and your health. This is your road to heal the body and to create a mutually supportive relationship so you can enjoy life to the maximum every single day. As in anything else in life, it is helpful to know what your final goal is and why it is important for you to reach your final vision.

The first step to improving your digestive health might seem completely irrelevant to digestion, as it has nothing to do with food, but it is essential to overall success.

chapter 15

YOUR WELLNESS VISION

A lbert Einstein said, "Imagination is everything. It is a preview of life's coming attractions."

You can't get to a happy future if you can't visualize what a happy future would entail for you. If you don't know where you want to go, how can you get there? You will feel lost if there is no direction.

One of the biggest mistakes most adults make is that they forget how to dream. They complain about their present circumstances, but they don't imagine their ideal world either. As kids, we daydream and imagine. As adults, we frown upon life's miseries and hope that someone in power will make our life better. So the biggest mistake is to not create dreams.

Creating an inspiring wellness vision is important! Just think about this quote from *Dream Manifesto*:[25]

> Think of it (vision) as ordering from the cosmic kitchen of the Universe. When you go into a restaurant, you don't want to tell the waiter that you want "food." Most of us are much more definite than that. In fact, we generally don't hesitate to tell the waiter exactly what we want, how we want it, and when we want it.

You have the power to bring forth into your life whatever you choose consciously. Think of your wellness vision as placing your order for health. Be clear about what you want and know that what you have ordered will be delivered.

Vision serves two goals:

- To inspire you to act in accordance with your values and goals. A personal vision that is based on values and beliefs that are important to you is the best motivator!

- To keep you focused on your desired future. It guides you through difficult decisions in life and through daily choices in food.

Creating vision is a combination of deep self-exploration and imagination. It is inspiring, reinvigorating, and exciting! You are creating your own future!

Your wellness vision should be based on your body and what feels good to you. Don't limit yourself to society's expectation of what health should be. If you listed a beautiful body or a flat, not bloated stomach in your vision, are you looking for a specific shape or a feeling of being comfortable in your own skin and being in love with yourself?

Here are some questions to think about while creating your wellness vision.

First, describe how it is now:

- How do you feel, physically? How is your digestion, your energy level, your body image, your relationship with your body?

Second, describe your ideal wellness vision:

Use at least three sentences to describe the way you feel about each of these aspects of your being.

- If you were at your optimum level of health and wellness, what would that look and feel like?
- How does your digestion function and make you feel?
- What do you feel when you see your body, and especially your stomach, in the mirror?
- What is your energy level like?
- How do you feel when you eat?
- How do you feel after you eat?
- How often do you go to the bathroom?

Clarity is everything! Make sure to write out your answers. If you take time in this section, your progress is going to be a lot faster and easier. If you skip this section and rush to the next chapter, you are likely to feel overwhelmed and stressed out by the to-do and not-to-do lists.

Some other helpful questions to think about:

- What is your biggest issue/problem/challenge connected to digestion?
- What is your biggest fear associated with it, if it is not resolved?
- What problem/symptoms would you like to solve or alleviate?
- How would you like to feel?

- Why does it truly matter to you to improve your digestion? (What is your motivation?)

- Why now?

- What will happen — or not happen — if you don't change and things keep going the way they are going now?

- What actions will you need to take to achieve this vision?

- What is your commitment to yourself for the time of healing?

- What will motivate you to keep taking daily action and sustain your vision?

- How confident are you that you will achieve this wellness vision?

- How committed are you to achieving your vision?

- What obstacles will you need to overcome to stay in action?

- What strategies will you use to overcome obstacles?

- In what ways will your life and relationships be enhanced by achieving your vision?

- What single step are you committed to taking today to begin walking toward your vision?

It might seem like a lot of questions, but please spend some time thinking about them and writing your answers. This is a major step in helping you move in the direction that you want. It will help you clarify your priorities and understand the WHY behind it, and it will keep you motivated throughout the whole process. There is nothing more inspirational than to review your wellness vision when you feel down, tired, and unmotivated to follow your healthy eating routine.

Following healthy rules that you decide to incorporate is not a matter of willpower alone; it is about staying connected to your ideal image of self, the state of being you would like to experience, living in integrity with your own values, and aligning your actions to support your values.

There is nothing better than a clear wellness vision and daily visualization to help with the creation of that internal alignment. A clear, inspiring vision helps to guide and support daily actions to be aligned with the vision itself. All of this goes back to living in alignment with your ideal vision of yourself. **If you know how you want to feel and look, you can choose foods and actions that will help you get there.** If you know that being feminine and graceful is one of your top goals, you can choose activities and foods that bring you closer to that state.

Only you can choose your diet to be nourishing and healing, not controlling and restricting, and your exercise to be fun and playful and not a battle with fat. The hardest part is doing what your body is telling you is the right thing to do and letting go of constantly comparing your diet and exercise regimen to others in the hope of finding something more effective.

Here is where the importance of having a clear wellness vision comes in. You need to have that bright picture of how you want to feel and look. Your wellness vision should be based on your values. It will guide you through the most difficult choices and change the most ingrained, unhealthy habits.

Your vision is your best support buddy in the times when you want to give up. Whenever you feel off track or start questioning your diet or exercise routine, do this little trick:

Come back to the ideal vision of yourself. See how you look and feel there. See yourself moving through your regular activities looking and feeling this way. Walking the streets, writing, working, interacting with people. Connect with that ideal picture of yourself. And then ask your ideal self what she does to feel that way. What she eats, what gets her inspired, what she enjoys doing for exercise. It will help to realign your daily actions with your ideal image.

If you get too busy to remember to reconnect to your vision on any given day, you will go back to relying on willpower. Willpower requires forcing things that with clear vision become inspired actions.

Once you have your vision in place, the next step is identifying behaviors that will help you get there. If you have habits that support your vision, achieving it is just a matter of time. If your current behaviors and habits are not aligned with your ideal vision of self, you will greatly benefit from doing some work around letting go of the old patterns.

So if you want to have a happy belly that digests food with ease and without making you feel five months pregnant, but currently you find yourself overeating at every other meal, you have to let go of this habit. If you want to go to the bathroom every morning without straining, but currently you eat mostly a gluten and dairy-based diet with very few greens, this pattern has to be replaced with a new one that supports your vision.

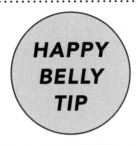

HAPPY BELLY TIP

Changing habits does not have to be overwhelming and 100 percent willpower-based. It is mostly about aligning your behaviors to your vision. You choose which behaviors and at what pace.

Once you decide on the new habits that you want to adopt and the old ones that you want to let go of, you will be able to create a weekly goal list to support your progress.

Before we get to the section on changing habits and SMART goal setting, I would like to share a part of my personal wellness vision. I hope it can serve as an example and inspiration.

Here is a piece of my personal vision:

I wake up without an alarm, rested, and feeling grateful. My body feels light and easy. My stomach is flat and feels light. I am full of calm, inspired energy and feel graceful in everything that I do. I am satisfied with small portions of nourishing high-quality food. I take time to eat slowly and mindfully. I take time to chew and to eat at the table. I listen to my body and trust it when it comes to eating and exercise. My body is wise and knows what it needs. We have a trusting and mutually supportive relationship. I pay attention to my body's signals and respect them. My stomach feels nourished, clean, and comfortable.

I feel confident and beautiful. I move with grace and lightness. I wear clothes that feel good on my body, and I feel comfortable in them. I exercise and rest enough. I treat myself with love and compassion. My digestion and energy are very strong.

My motivators/my WHY

I deserve to feel healthy and to be full of energy every day, to feel confident and happy in my body. I need to feel clear and inspired to do the work I am meant to do. It is important for me to live in integrity with my values and in accordance with what I teach and write about, to inspire my students, to be at peace with myself.

Here is an example of a vision that one of my clients decided to share publicly to inspire others: http://www.spinachandyoga.com/living-a-dream/.

Before skipping to the next section, write out your own wellness vision around your digestion and health in general. Write it out in detail so it comes alive when you think about it. The more you connect with it, the more powerful its effect will be.

chapter 16

KEY COMPONENTS OF HEALING

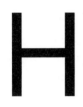ere are the key components of healing at a glance:

- willingness to commit to creating a trusting, compassion-based relationship with your body and your digestion.

- willingness to create a dialogue with your body and start listening to what it needs.

- willingness to commit to a journey, not short-term changes.

- willingness to take full responsibility for how you feel in your body.

- willingness to learn to and adopt good eating habits and include more easy-to-digest foods.

- willingness to let go of habits that don't serve you and your body.

- willingness to let go of thoughts and beliefs that are hurting your body.

- willingness to create a healing space in your kitchen and/ or dining room.

- willingness to add nourishing, healing self-care into daily life.

- willingness to engage in the practice of daily mindfulness to make the change easier.

- willingness to focus daily on how you want to feel or look, not focus on, or dread, things you dislike.

SELF-TRUST

Before jumping to making changes, cleaning out your kitchen cupboards, and dropping gluten, dairy, and all the bad eating habits at once, stop! Change doesn't have to be overwhelming. It has to be smart and based on your individual needs.

Before pinpointing the areas that need work, you need to become really honest with yourself. Your readiness to take the cover-up off and get real will, in a big way, determine your success.

Now that you know what habits and foods can hinder digestion, it's time to reevaluate your current habits, tendencies, thoughts around food, and emotions related to eating and your digestion. Our goal is to identify the biggest culprits on your road to a healthy digestion and a flat stomach without chronic bloating, constipation, or persistent heartburn.

Getting honest can be challenging. We all tend to under-report the amount of food we eat, over-report the amount of movement we engage in, and in general, avoid recognizing mistakes. Awareness of mistakes brings out negative emotions and guilt. In this case, it shouldn't! You will not be judging yourself for your bad behaviors or poor food choices, or for not following a set of rules.

An attitude of compassion and vulnerability is the only way to re-create trust between body and mind. For most of us, there is not a lot of trust between these two life-long partners. Trust has been broken too many times through unkept promises, unmet goals, and unrealized dreams. How many times has our mind set a goal to avoid sugar or bread just to find the body eating a bag of cookies two days later?

You wouldn't trust your partner if he promised to keep his hands off other women only to be found at your girlfriend's apartment, would you? So quite possibly, your mind doesn't trust your body to collaborate, and your body thinks of your mind as a controlling, abusive freak.

To change this negative, mutually abusive relationship, it is important to be honest with yourself and evaluate your state of affairs. Where does the relationship between your body and your mind stand right now? What are their expectations from each other? Does your mind expect your body to go, go, go, without a break on no sleep and without fresh food? Does your body feel betrayed and tired?

See, our mind-body relationship is very similar to any relationship. Without trust, there is no basis for a healthy relationship. If you think your partner can beat you up, cheat on you, or torture you at any moment, you just won't be committed to that relationship. Imagine being stuck with a partner who abuses you. This is how our body feels. Our body doesn't have a choice of whom it gets as an owner/partner. Our mind-body relationship is the only truly lifelong relationship we will ever have. Nevertheless, we spend very little time making sure that this relationship is a loving and a happy one.

We can easily torture our body by feeding it poorly chewed, hard-to-digest, processed food. Without paying attention to its feelings, we make it sit all day without movement. We poison it with drugs and alcohol or torture it at the gym with draining workouts—all this without ever asking for forgiveness. And it still tries to support us and function the best it can. If you feel that your internal relationship is not where you would like it to be, you can change it, starting right now.

CREATE INNER DIALOGUE: WHAT IS YOUR BODY TELLING YOU?

Your body is not your enemy. It wants to feel good, be healthy, and have energy. It naturally strives to be in balance. We just don't always listen to it and don't always support it.

At one point or another, most of us feel that our body is slowing down our progress to live our dreams, or that it gets in the way. It might be the whole body or just one particular area.

> If it weren't for my bloated stomach, I would be able to wear my favorite sexy dress and finally find the love of my life. If it weren't for my chunky legs, I would be so much more desirable and attractive. If it weren't for my stretch marks, I would have an amazing sex life. If it weren't for my big nose, I would be the happiest person in the world. Why does my stomach have to be so sensitive and require so much attention to food?

Do you have thoughts similar to the ones above about any particular organ or part of your body?

Emotionally, we send a lot of negative energy to that part of the body. We reject it, curse it, blame it, struggle with it. We don't want to accept it, love it, caress it, or take care of it.

We also get caught up in the "if only/I would" mode, in jealousy toward people who have it "better" and "easier," and in trying to "fix" things.

When something is painful or unpleasant, we tend to avoid feeling it as much as possible. It's a natural response. I've noticed that most women who suffer from bloating don't breathe into their belly. They try to avoid feeling that area. A lot of women who are unhappy with their weight wear baggy, ugly clothes that don't flatter them in any way but instead hide the so-called imperfections. Similarly, people who hate their insomnia or anxiety take pills to mask the symptoms, refusing to experience those unpleasant feelings.

This desire to "fix" as quickly as possible and avoid feeling bad, unfortunately, often stops us from learning from our body. Every unpleasant feeling, symptom, disease, is a way for our body to communicate and tell us something useful about our environment, relationships, behaviors, food, or emotional patterns. Feeling bad is a sign that we need to learn something. Unless you actively try to understand the lesson, this bad feeling and the pattern that creates it will keep reoccurring.

The only way to understand the lesson that our wise body is trying to share is to be present and listen. It means accepting the present situation, acknowledging it, and observing the way your body feels.

It also might mean taking responsibility for bringing on that symptom and asking your body for forgiveness and guidance in making things better. Your body is not against you; it is on your team. It's your best partner and teacher. The more you listen, are present with whatever is, the more your body will share. Its voice will get easier to understand, and you will trust it more.

An area of your body or an organ that might be causing distress or negativity in your life needs attention, love, and support. A bloated belly needs a cup of hot herbal tea with ginger and fennel, not an angry voice of judgment. Tired adrenals need rest and relaxation, not caffeine. Anxiety might need a warm oil massage and a hot bath with essential oil, candles, and soothing music over prescription medication.

As you can see, what I am talking about is creating more internal dialogue with your body, more listening to your body, creating a love and care-based relationship with each organ and your body as a whole. It might not be easy to love and accept a digestive system that keeps you on a strict diet, or a diseased liver that makes you sensitive to fats and alcohol, or an insomnia that makes you tired and groggy. But struggling with your own body is worse. Through accepting and choosing love and attention, we can create positive change or at least live with more peace and calm.

You can treat your symptoms as if they were pleading for help, not as if they are an unwelcome annoyance in your life. So if your stomach feels bloated and heavy, try looking at it as a message from your body that the past meal (or the way it was eaten) is not fostering vibrant health. I would say something like this to myself: "Thank you, body, for letting me learn this lesson. I hear you and I understand you. I know that what and how I eat determines the state of my health and energy. I will do my best to support you in the future. I will also be more careful with this type of food. Forgive me for causing you discomfort. How can I help you deal with it better?"

This is very different from what I would have said to myself a few years ago! And you don't have to repeat exactly the same words. Your dialogue with your body might be very different. Just experiment with it and do it daily. As in any relationship, the relationship between ourselves and our body takes daily attention, patience, trust, and compassion.

The next time you feel bad, unpleasant, stuck, bloated, heavy, or anything else negative, before masking the symptoms, take five minutes to be present with those feelings. Be with your cravings, be with your pain, be with your discomfort—just BE. Ask your body what it is trying to communicate to you through this pain. What is the lesson here?

The more you breathe into WHAT IS, the more likely the lesson will become clear and the discomfort will dissolve. Once your body knows that you are listening, it will stop trying to get your attention with dramatic measures. It will communicate with gentler and pleasanter sensations.

Robin Lee is an alternative medicine practicioner and the founder of www.intuitionheals.com. I was lucky enough to have a session with Robin and do an interview on listening to what our bodies say. Robin says, "Our bodies are incredibly happy to communicate with us; we just need to remember to slow down and make it a priority to listen. The biggest trick to learning to connect to yourself is making the space, asking a question, taking a breath and time to listen—and then honoring what your body has requested you do to support it."

It can be strange to start including your body in making decisions about your health and giving it authority, but in the end it works, so who cares if it is strange?

Your Turn

Now take time to ask your body, your belly, what it is trying to share. What would it ask from you to help with healing? Which habits or behaviors are hurting it? What creates all the digestive discomfort and pain that you have to deal with? What do you have to say to your belly?

If you are serious about helping your body heal, take some time every single day to talk to your body, to check in with it. It might take time to hear the answers, but they will come. If you haven't had a dialogue between your body and yourself in a long time, the exercise below will be helpful in starting it.

LOVE LETTER TO YOUR BODY—ONE SIMPLE EXERCISE TO BUILD A BETTER RELATIONSHIP WITH YOURSELF!

For many of us it is difficult to create a dialogue with our body if we haven't talked to it for our entire lifetime. The exercise that I describe below is one of the best ways to start building that dialogue.

You write kind messages and e-mails to your loved ones, friends, family, and everyone that you care about. They deserve to know that you care about them and love them. Sharing your feelings is what makes the relationship stronger. How would you like to live with someone who never tells you that he cares about you or loves you? No matter how open we are with others, we rarely communicate openly with ourselves. Nobody ever told us that we need to.

Have you ever thought of writing a love letter to your body — your dear body that you've been living with for your entire life, your patient body that you spend every moment of the day and night with?

Through the good and bad times, your body never left you, never betrayed you, was always there for you.

I bet you can remember the last time you gave a compliment to another person but would have a harder time recollecting a compliment to yourself.

It is time to correct it!

When I work with my clients, we talk a lot about body confidence, body and mind relationship, and ways to improve it. A LOVE LETTER exercise is one of the techniques that many women find almost life changing. It gives them a new perspective and a new level of inspiration to change old patterns of behavior that might be hurting their body.

Here is a love letter written by one of the participants. It is touching, emotional, raw, and honest. Read it. And then write your own!

Dear Body,

I want you to know that I continue to be amazed by your strength and resilience. For the past 18 years, now half of your life, you have tolerated constant abuse. You have stood strong for 12-hour shifts in over 100-degree kitchens, bending, lifting and carrying heavy, hot items. In all of that time, you never let me down.

I repaid you for all of your hard work with burns and cuts on a regular basis, many late nights spent overindulging on fatty foods and alcohol, and never enough rest.

There was also the time when I put you through painful procedures and pumped you up with unnatural hormones prescribed by doctors. I should have been a better advocate for you, insisting on a more thorough answer instead of a quick fix. I should have invested time in a better solution.

There is some good news too. You are blessed to be loved by someone. This wonderful, generous man has encouraged you to take a break and rest.

I hope it is not too late, but I would like a chance to make it up to you. I have used this time to get us back on a routine of exercise, which will make you stronger and ultimately happier. I have learned to listen to what you need, and will feed you accordingly. So much of my life has been spent feeding others, and neglecting you. The time has come to focus on healthful, nutritious meals.

I still have scars, so I will never forget all that you have already done for me. We have many beautiful years left together, and I am committed to treating you with love and kindness. I am grateful for our journey, and looking forward to the future.

Love, Me

Your Turn

For this exercise to be effective, reading another person's letter is not enough; you need to write your own. Before reading any further, take a notebook or open your laptop and write a love letter to your body. If you feel inspired, you can write a response letter from your body to you. For the dialogue to start, you need to initiate it, because your body has been told to shut up too many times. Now it is your turn to speak and then invite your body to speak back to you.

SET YOUR MIND FOR A JOURNEY, NOT A DESTINATION

Improving health is a journey. Maintaining health is a journey of its own. Living in a stressful, polluted, fast-changing world, our bodies' needs change, and we must continuously keep learning and implementing that knowledge in daily life.

I can't promise you that this healing journey will be easy or fast, but if you are committed to creating integrity and commitment in your relationship with your body, if you are willing to re-create trust with yourself and your instincts (gut), and to recognize and analyze the behaviors that might be hurting your body and your soul, you will be creating better health.

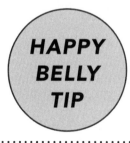

HAPPY BELLY TIP

Create an agreement with yourself and commit to act out of kindness and improvement of mind and body relationship, not just until you feel better but for the rest of your life.

Eating food is one of the most important activities that will determine the relationship between your body and your mind. Through your eating, you can see if there is integrity in that relationship, if it is full of trust and love, or if it subsists on self-abuse and disrespect. Through this relationship you can create dramatic shifts. You can reclaim the relationship between your mind and body and make it nourishing, loving, and based on integrity and compassion. When you eat to nourish your lifelong partner (your body) it will be easier to stay mindful of your body's cues. You will know what to eat and when to stop intuitively without anyone telling you. Your mind doesn't know how much food is enough, but your body does. You must listen to your body to obtain this knowledge. If you don't do this, you will spend your entire life searching for a miracle prescription of what to eat and how much to eat, and most likely will always have to rely on willpower and control, not self-love and trust. In my opinion, living your entire life in a controlling relationship is not the best way to spend your life.

Life gets busy, things get noisy, and it might be hard to hear your internal voice telling you that you don't need that cookie to feel good. When we ignore that voice, even for a minute, old behavior patterns can reemerge and take over. This journey will never end. It might become easier with time, but it will keep rolling while we are alive.

TAKE RESPONSIBILITY

As Lissa Rankin, MD, carefully noted in her book *Mind over Medicine*, we are brought up in a culture in which doctors are supposed to carry the responsibility of creating and maintaining a healthy society.[26] They are supposed to know what it takes to keep us healthy and well. The main flaw of this perception is that it is based on the theory that doctors know your body better than you do and that your body is exactly the same as your coworker's, your mother's, your trainer's, or your partner's.

Only that is not the case. Nobody knows more about your situation and about your body than you do. Most doctors don't have time to learn everyone's life story. But everything that happened to you throughout your life will have an effect on your current needs and best treatments. It might seem like a tempting solution to hand over the reins of your health to someone who has more knowledge and who does it for a living. Taking responsibility for your own health is quite a load to carry. It means more decisions, more thinking for yourself, more listening to your body. Why would you want that when you can just go to the doctor and get your solution—albeit temporary and with a lot of side effects—within minutes?

It might seem daunting to take this huge responsibility for how you feel, but at the same time, it is empowering, and in reality, it is your only hope to create a vibrant, healthy life. You can't argue with the fact that every single action that you take has a butterfly effect on your health. Overeating for dinner tonight is very likely to lead to a puffy face, a bloated stomach and low energy tomorrow. This is a choice that you make and how you feel is the result of this choice. You can choose to feel vibrant, light, and healthy, or heavy, bloated, and constipated.

Your body has an innate ability to heal and balance itself. You just need to allow it and to help it when needed.

HAPPY BELLY TIP

To heal and stay in balance, we must remember that it is our responsibility to nurture and support our bodies the best that we possibly can in any given moment.

COMMIT TO NURTURING SELF-CARE

As an incredibly committed partner, our body tries its best to love and support us no matter what. It keeps on pushing through. It keeps on surviving until, one day, it just can't anymore. And then we start feeling drained, tired, sick, bloated, constipated, fat, and drowned in self-pity and self-hate.

We are our own enemies. We abuse our bodies and digestive system almost every day. The body doesn't have a voice; it can't tell us what to do. It can't complain to the police or call 911. It has to quietly put up with us, find ways to recover, and keep working until it BREAKS DOWN.

Even if we think that we live the healthiest lifestyle possible considering the circumstances, it is almost impossible not to engage in regular body abuse if we live in a modern society. What matters is the degree of abuse, the awareness of the fact that you are hurting your body, and what we do to heal the negative effects.

Some regular day-to-day things can be pretty abusive and disruptive to all internal organs, particularly digestion. See how many you check off.

- ☐ not sleeping enough
- ☐ working out when you are tired
- ☐ not moving your body for days or weeks at a time
- ☐ drinking coffee/taking stimulants when tired instead of taking a break
- ☐ drinking energy drinks to work out "harder" or stay up when tired

- ☐ overeating

- ☐ not eating enough

- ☐ overexercising to the point of exhaustion because more is better

- ☐ eating while walking or standing

- ☐ not checking in to see how your body and stomach feel

- ☐ breathing very shallow and fast

- ☐ not eating enough nutrient-dense foods

- ☐ treating symptoms without resolving the root cause

- ☐ eating nonfood items made out of chemicals

- ☐ eating foods that don't digest well

- ☐ bingeing on food or alcohol

- ☐ eating when upset or bored

- ☐ not eating when hungry

- ☐ not going to the bathroom regularly

- ☐ ignoring the body's urges for the sake of being polite to others

Many of us are guilty of at least some of the above.

To stay well and healthy, your body and your gut need love and a commitment to life-force-giving, healing activities and healthy foods. As in any relationship, you and your body need to learn how to live together and enjoy life without abuse and power struggles.

A huge part of healing this relationship is to focus on self-care. Food is an important aspect of it. You can eat to nourish your body, or use your body purely as a vehicle to experience pleasure. When you eat a cookie, you are not doing it to meet the needs of your body, you are doing it selfishly to experience pleasure. You don't care if it will hurt you. You just want a few seconds of a sweet bliss.

I believe that truly nourishing food has to be delightful both to the body and the mind. Purely functional eating for nutrients and vitamins would turn us into robots. A nourishing way of eating is about eating foods that are easy to digest and make you fully satiated both physically and emotionally.

Although eating nourishing, easy-to-digest foods is one of the self-care components, there is much more to it. Deep regular relaxation, deep breathing, nourishing movement, sunshine, fresh air, play, massage, a fulfilling sex life, time alone to recharge, occasional retreats to contemplate, and connection with other people are all important aspects of self-care. We will discuss some of them in this book shortly, but please explore each one of them on your own and make time every day for self-care.

···

chapter 17

OPTIMIZING INNATE HEALING ABILITY

A key to optimizing most functions in the body is a calm nervous system—a relaxed state of being. Digestion is no exception. Our body is able to handle even diffi-cult-to-digest foods, complicated food combinations, and less-than-ideal ingredients a lot more efficiently when we are not stressed.

I feel it a lot and always think of the relaxation effect as a "vacation state of being." When you are comfortable, enjoying the moment, not in a rush, and focusing on doing enjoyable things for yourself, your body happily resets into a healthier mode.

One of the first things I learned when I was a teenager interested in yoga was that yoga done in a mindful, slow-paced way helps to elicit a relaxation response, which is necessary to turn on the self-healing mechanisms of the body. Relaxation is a prerequisite for our body to start fixing things. When we are in a stress-induced fight-or-flight response, our body is prepared to run, fight, or climb a tree, but not to rest, digest, and heal. For the self-repairing mechanism to turn on, we need to feel safe. We need to feel relaxed. Unfortunately, for a lot of people this deep relaxation never occurs, even at night.

According to Dana James, the founder of Food Coach NYC, who was mentioned in the section on food sensitivities, stress, with its fight or flight response, has a very detrimental effect on our gut. Eventually perpetual stress response can lead to leaky gut and multiple food sensitivities. Food sensitivities in turn lead to unpleasant digestive symptoms such as gas, bloating, food-related fatigue, low-grade inflammation, and constipation.

Lissa Rankin covered the negative effects of a constant stress response at length in her book *Mind Over Medicine*. She also mentioned that it is necessary to initiate physiological relaxation to turn on the body's self-repair mechanisms to repair digestion or any other organ in the body. It is the opposite of the fight-or-flight response that we have during most waking hours if we live in a big city, have a busy job, and are taking care of a family. Continuous showering of the body's internal organs with adrenaline and cortisol can eventually be manifested in indigestion, bloating, cramps, and other unpleasant symptoms.

When we elicit a relaxation response, our blood chemistry changes, stress hormones drop, health-inducing hormones are released, and the parasympathetic nervous system takes over. When the parasympathetic nervous system is active, our body is in a state of digesting and healing. Our body needs to be rested to have the energy to heal, whether it is healing and optimizing digestion or healing any other body part.

If you break your leg and put a cast on it and start taking supplements to help with healing, but won't stop walking on it, it will take a lot longer to heal. If you reduce the stress load on the leg and rest, your body will do the job of healing rather quickly.

It works very similarly with digestion. If you are rested and relaxed, your body can digest and heal the irritation in the gut. Puffiness from the inflammation will go down and the energy level will go up if the stress hormones are reduced.

While it would be ideal to take a few weeks at a spa to heal the gut, I realize it is not realistic for most of us to take a vacation after each meal. What we can learn to do is create a "vacation" frame of mind, a relaxed state of being.

When you are relaxed, your entire body softens and feels easy and expansive. Stress on the other hand feels tight, constrictive, and difficult. Once you know what relaxation feels like in your body, you will be able to re-create it on demand. It is an incredibly powerful skill that can reduce the negative effect of stressful events that happen throughout the day.

A SOFT APPROACH TO STRICT RULES

When you make a decision for yourself that you would like to feel better and that you are ready to improve your relationship with your body through internal dialogue, self-care, and creating habits around foods that help your body thrive, you need to create change in a soft, not stress-inducing way.

You already have enough stress in your life. Adding more to it with strict dietary restrictions, a must-do daily self-care checklist, and a three-page supplement list can trigger quite a bit of stress if approached in a militant way. Your perspective on your actions will determine whether you add more stress or if you allow your nervous system to relax, your "matrix to soften" (as Dr. Claudia Welch, the author of *Balance Your Hormones, Balance Your Life*[27] says), and your actions to stem from self-love and compassion. From my mentors, friends, and clients I have learned that self-care should be done from a place of love, of gratitude, not as another task that stresses you out on your to-do list. Healing digestion is an act of self-care toward your body. Eating healing foods, engaging in relaxing nourishing activities, listening to music that makes you feel alive, using spices, teas, or supplements are all examples of self-care.

Perspective on your digestion-healing protocol will, in large part, determine your success. A lot of women feel extremely restricted when hard-to-digest, irritating foods are off the menu grid. As soon as this happens, an internal war starts between mind and body. The mind says that the only road to a flat stomach and a regular digestion is through a gluten- and dairy-free diet, and the body that is used to a certain way of eating resists with every cell.

Wouldn't you want to make the healing a bit more peaceful? It is an opportunity to really get mind and body to feel that they are a part of one team, moving toward the same goals. Instead of telling yourself that you are going on a strict diet, frame it in a more compassionate way: "I am committing to nourish my body with healing, easy-to-digest foods for the next . . . (period of time). It is my time to reconnect with my body and to help it heal so we can enjoy life to the fullest."

Restriction versus two months of immense self-love—which one would you choose? Which one would you stick to longer? Which one would bring more pleasure? Which one would be more likely to activate a relaxing and self-healing mode in your nervous system?

If you focus on what you are doing and including, instead of what you are avoiding or banning from your life and diet, your body will respond very differently.

Eating good-quality, nourishing food in a relaxed environment is an act of kindness to your body, and of self-love. Stuffing down a deli sandwich (even a gluten-free one) while walking is an act of self-abuse, and it makes the relationship between your body and mind tense and filled with distrust.

If you commit to healing your digestion through the practice of self-love and compassion for a day, what would it look like for you?

THE NECESSITY OF COUCH TIME FOR HEALING

Your approach to creating new habits and diet should not induce a stress response. The rest of your life should focus on keeping your body in a state that is optimal for the healing and digestion to occur.

Each one of us can find her own favorite ways to reduce stress and induce a relaxed state of being that optimizes healing and digestion. It can be a daily practice that you do before dinner, or a breathing technique that you do every time your breath becomes too shallow, or a phrase that you repeat to yourself in traffic. There is no right or wrong here. It is best to try several and stick with the ones that work for you. As long as you do it consistently and feel its softening, relaxing effect, you are golden!

Below are a few stress-reducing techniques that have worked for my clients and me and that you can try for yourself. Books have been written about each one, so this is just a short introduction.

MINDFUL BREATHING

One of the fastest ways to relax and reconnect to your body is through mindful breathing. Most women don't even realize how shallow their breath is. We also don't pay attention to all the times when we hold our breath during stressful moments. When we are not breathing fully, we don't feel our body.

The most ingenious, effective things are usually very simple. When we learn them and see how effective they are firsthand, we usually say: "Really? I can't believe it's so simple!" Deep breathing is one of those things. We all want to feel light and at ease in our body. Who doesn't like that pleasant feeling of soft, relaxed shoulders; a relaxed jaw; an open chest that allows every breath to flow freely; a happy, satisfied belly that easily expands and softens with every breath; joints that feel nicely lubricated and free to move; muscles that create flowing, graceful movement? You can see people who feel this way in their body right away in any crowd. They stand out. They seem tall, graceful; they have energy that says, "grounded but light, relaxed yet strong, centered yet very open." They glow. They never seem to be in a rush. Things come easily to them. Worry and anxiety seem not to exist in their lives.

There is one thing that helps to bring me closer to feeling this way. Every time I practice it consistently for a few days, it completely shifts my day. It creates more flow and less friction, more ease and less tightness.

This simple thing is SO-HUM breathing. Dr. Vasant Lad, the founder of the Ayurvedic Institute, often refers to so-hum breathing as the most powerful health and spiritual practice.

It is simple. You don't need any equipment. It doesn't cost a penny, and it takes just a few minutes to learn. One of the best things is that you can do it anywhere, even while you are busy.

So-hum is the natural sound of our breath. To do so-hum breathing, sit comfortably on a pillow or chair. You can also lie down or practice this breathing while walking. Bring your attention to the breath.

Consciously trace the breath moving through your entire body. If there are any points of tension, relax them. Let your stomach and chest move freely with every breath. Then, mentally start pronouncing "SO" on the inhale and "HUM" on the exhale. With every breath, let those words be your only focus. Listen to your own breath and those words in your mind. After a few breaths, it should feel very natural, as if the body is making SO-HUM sounds on its own.

Don't force your breath; just let it flow effortlessly. Be an observer for a while. Let the lungs open up and breathe deeply without any rush. Deep diaphragmatic breathing activates the parasympathetic nervous system, which counters the body's fight-or-flight response to stress and puts us in rest-and-digest mode instead. Bring your attention to the sensation of the breath flowing in and out of your nostrils. This will keep your mind from wandering. Keep doing it for five minutes to begin with, and then you can do it for as long as you want whenever you want. This is the beauty of breathing—there are no tools or space required. Just you and your body.

MEDITATION

Meditation is scientifically proven to induce a relaxation response and to reduce stress. It also improves resistance to stress, so it works not only while you are doing it but after you are finished too. Cardiologist Herbert Benson studied the effects of meditation on multiple disorders including allergic skin reactions, depression, anxiety, infertility, ulcers, fatigue, postoperative swelling, PMS, abdominal pain, and other conditions. Meditation is found to counterbalance the fight-or-flight response in the body and promote self-healing mechanisms.

Meditation is not just for yogis and it doesn't have to be boring! Meditation is different for everyone. Choose the type of meditation that makes you feel your best. You can choose to do a guided relaxation/meditation, enjoy a 10-minute yoga nidra (yogic sleep), do "loving kindness" meditation, or practice with any YouTube video or smartphone application that feels right for you. Your goal is to feel relaxed, inspired, and to enjoy the activity. Whatever you choose to do, focus on being in the present, being aware of your body, your surroundings, and your breath.

Never meditate as if you were doing another nagging task. As one of my favorite authors and teachers, Dr. Claudia Welch, says, "Meditate with love toward yourself, your body, and those around you." Try to cultivate feelings of being "in love" and of gratitude when you meditate. Feeling "in love" is one of the strongest techniques to reverse the negative effects of stress on your body.

Paul Brunton, a philosopher and a writer, describes the effects of meditation on one's life in a very beautiful way: "Life becomes spacious and unstrained, its horizon of daily living enlarged, when a still timelessness creeps into a man's make-up. He will become less hurried but not less active. He knows that his future is assured because his present conduct is serene and that it is safe because his present understanding is right."[28]

Even a short morning meditation helps you realign to the wellness vision and to the feelings that you want to experience in your daily life. Every single day you may want to connect to the feeling of having regular, healthy digestion that works with ease and efficiency. Your body will know what to do throughout the day to help you get there.

Meditation is a way to recharge your battery and to create inspired actions throughout the day that will help bring you closer to your vision one day at a time. It is one of the only ways to choose inspiration over motivation and willpower when it comes to changing habits.

I find that visualization is an easier way to start a meditation practice for many people. We are used to keeping our brain busy. So, emptying it and stopping all the thoughts is not easy in the beginning. In my experience, you can't force meditation; it just happens when you are ready. You can use various techniques to help prepare, but there is no benefit in rushing or forcing it.

Visualization is a great stepping stone to prepare for meditation. It is also a great tool to initiate healing on a subconscious level. It is helpful in fostering new habits in a nonforceful way through feeling connected and inspired. I recorded a special Happy Belly guided visualization for you. You can download it for free at www. spinachandyoga.com/resources.

You might be thinking: "I am too busy to meditate." It is similar to saying, "I'm in a rush, but I don't have time to look for car keys, so I'll just walk." Taking a few minutes out of your day to slow down and give your busy mind a break will make you more efficient in everything else you do. This time investment pays back really well in health and productivity.

Meditation can be very helpful in clearing negative thought patterns and raising your vibration. When you feel happy, you heal faster, and you treat your body better.

GET ENOUGH SLEEP AND TAKE NAPS

This one seems straightforward, but nevertheless, it never hurts to remind yourself that sleep is healing. Sleep recharges your inner batteries, your innate sense of peace and well-being, and provides time for the body to perform essential housekeeping. During the day, you are busy spending stored energy as well as digesting and assimilating today's food for tomorrow's energy. At night, your body performs important internal maintenance while you rest in an inactive state. It is a time for internal transformation, tissue regeneration, and purification.

WALK IN NATURE

Walking in nature is one of the easiest ways to reconnect to the five elements that make up the whole universe and your body. Leave your phone at home and get outside at least on the weekend. Instead of paying attention to your Facebook feed, spend some time resting your eyes on the green leaves and grass. Your body will recharge both physically and mentally.

REPEATING OF A PHRASE/ PRAYER/ OR MANTRA

Dr. Herbert Benson, in his bestselling book *The Relaxation Response*,[29] studied the effect of repeating a phrase or a word on the mental and emotional state. According to his research, it significantly helped to reduce the stress response and initiate relaxation.

You might think it's a bit woo-woo, but don't disregard anything before trying it. Logic and research junkie that I am, I started looking for an explanation behind the mantra magic. Why would a set of different words repeated over and over have a stress-reducing effect?

According to *A Harvard Medical School Special Health Report: Stress Management—Approaches for Preventing and Reducing Stress*: "The relaxation response triggered by a repetition of a simple phrase or a word leads to a body-wide slowdown and a feeling of well-being that have measurably positive effects on disorders caused by stress or made worse by it, including high blood pressure, abnormal heart rhythms, and many digestive disorders."[30]

You can use any simple word, mantra, or phrase. Dr. Benson is not picky about the words themselves. Any technique from any tradition, religious or secular, in his opinion, will do. But he emphasizes that you have to do it every day to get the benefits.

All you need to do is choose one word or phrase and repeat it single-mindedly for 10–15 minutes a day, or when you feel anxious, worried, or stressed. If other thoughts come to your mind, just gently bring your attention back to your words.

Words that might be good to try are: om, so-hum, shanti, peace, love, one, I am one, I am well, I forgive, thank you.

If you try it, *commit to doing it at least for a week every day* and at the end of the week *take a note of your current emotional state*. Think of it as an experiment—no expectations, just honest evaluation.

MASSAGE AWAY STRESS

Relaxing warm-oil massages can help reduce IBS symptoms if they are stress-related.

Massage is probably one of the most pleasant, stress-reducing, craving-fighting, nervous-system-pacifying activities there is.[31]

Studies show that massage therapy can increase the body's output of endorphins and serotonin, chemicals that act as natural painkillers and mood regulators. At the same time, massage also reduces the levels of cortisol, the hormone that might be responsible for irritable bowel and other types of digestive unease.

If you have time and resources, you can always get a massage at a spa. However, making it fancy is not necessary to get the benefits. A short, 15-minute shoulder or foot massage at a nail salon works as well. It is also more affordable, both time-wise and money-wise, so you can do it more often.

My favorite, though, is a pre-bedtime two- to three-minute foot massage with coconut oil (summer) or sesame oil (winter). I keep oil next to my bed so it is easy to remember. Every night, I take a bit, warm it up in my palms, and gently rub it on my feet, legs, and arms. It is a perfectly soothing and very calming practice. It helps me fall asleep faster, shows my body that I care about it, and helps to shift my nervous system into a peaceful rest-and-digest state.

When you are calm, you have a lot more understanding of what your body needs in terms of food, and you will be less likely to overeat or give in to emotional eating.

You can use coconut oil, sesame oil, or almond oil for a prebed-time foot massage. Keep the oil near the bed. As soon as you see it, you will remember why it is there. It makes creating a new habit very easy.

It might seem as if it doesn't have much to do with digestion, but in reality, emotional eating, overeating, and bingeing are all part of a stress response or an inability to deal with stress. Purely physiological changes in stomach acid and enzyme secretion are also directly related to stress. Improving digestion is not only about the food that you eat. Sometimes taking care of your nervous system might have more of a positive impact than eating only veggies.

chapter 18

CREATE A HEALING ENVIRONMENT

Your environment matters!

Look at all the areas of your life and analyze them for similarities of what is happening with your body and particularly with your digestion. Your health often reflects your environment. Unconsciously, the state of your relationship, work, clutter at home, and so on, can all show up in your health.

Does your closet look like a bloated mess? Do you have useless things stuck all around your house? Does thinking about your work make you feel constricted and tense, not in the flow?

Come back to your wellness vision now and add a few lines about how the house or apartment of your ideal self looks. What other areas of your life are not aligned with your ideal vision of self? Let yourself be fully immersed in that vision so, for the time being, you know exactly how you feel and what you do to feel that way.

To read my story of how I reevaluated my environment and how that helped me heal my digestive issues and polycystic ovarian syndrome go to www.spinachandyoga.com/environment.

Your Turn

Look at all areas of your life and see if a pattern emerges. Is there something similar between what you feel in your stomach and what you feel about the outside world? Do you let yourself digest the events and emotions? Are you holding stuff in? Are you overspending, overcluttering, and overeating?

Awareness is the first step to creating a change. What you notice might first upset you, but it will also help you get clear on what needs to change. It is said, "The truth will set you free. But first, it's going to piss you off." Practice nonjudgmental awareness of your environment and create change for the better.

chapter 19

THE MAGIC OF POSITIVE THOUGHTS

"Whatever we focus on grows!" If we focus on the positive, there will be more of it appearing in our life. Unfortunately, it is true with the negative thoughts as well. That's the way positive psychology explains this phenomenon.

Modern neuroscientists, working in the field of positive psychology, have been able to prove that our attitude and perception have a strong impact on reality. Our brain will rewire the entire body to make it correspond to our current beliefs. So if we believe that we are overweight, it will be so; if we are certain that we are getting old quickly, we might. On the other hand, if we think that our body is strong and beautiful, our body will respond to that belief as well. For those with a critical mindset, here is a glimpse at some of the science.

In 1981, a Harvard study led by Ellen Langer placed men in their 70s and 80s in the simulated 1950s. The environment was re-created with magazines, radio stations with programs from that era, movies, games, and conversations. Everything was done to trick the brain into thinking that it was living in the '50s. In a week, psychologists compared prestudy and poststudy memory, intelligence, hearing, vision, and flexibility of the participating seniors. The poststudy results impressed even the scientists. Those men seemed to have gotten younger.[32]

This study provided evidence for a simple but invaluable fact: wherever we put the mind, the body will follow. It is not our physical state that limits us; it is our mindset about our own limits—our perceptions—that draws the line.

Lissa Rankin, in her bestselling book *Mind over Medicine*, describes a few amazing cases of the placebo effect, which is basically the effect of belief on the body. When people believe that they are getting an effective medicine, they get better. The *Journal of Clinical Investigation* described a patient who suffered from severe nausea and vomiting due to a chaotic pattern of contractions in the stomach. In the study, she was offered a new, magical, extremely potent drug, which doctors promised would cure her nausea. Within minutes, the patient felt better and her stomach contractions were normal. The only thing is that doctors gave her ipecac, not a new miracle drug. Ipecac actually induces vomiting. The nauseated patient just really believed that the medicine would make her better, and it did![33]

This case, along with many similar ones, proves that what happens in our mind could have a strong effect on the body. In drug studies, about a third of patients, after taking sugar or salt water, usually have physiological changes that improve their symptoms or completely cure them, according to Dr. Henry Beecher, writing in the *Journal of the American Medical Association*.[34]

As Lissa Rankin interestingly notes, that placebo doesn't just change the way we *feel*; it actually creates physiological changes in the body. Colon inflammation decreases, blood pressure becomes lower, and the chemistry of our blood changes.

So what if the beliefs that you have about food and supplements have more of an effect on your digestive health than the food itself?

Imagine someone who considers that she is doing her body good by eating an eight-grain cereal mix with nuts and raisins for breakfast. Then she has a guest stay over, and that guest just read that grains can be rough on digestion, that they can cause irritation, and help grow candida. Which one of these people will feel better after they eat the cereal? One eats with gratitude for having an opportunity to nourish her body with good food, and the other eats with fear, expecting something negative to happen in her body.

Our body responds to what we think and expect. You need to feel good about the food choices that you make. If we eat with a fear that the food is not good for us, if we expect to feel bad after something, these thoughts will bring those feelings into reality.

When you are in a situation in which the food choice is limited, focus on the good aspects of the food that you have in front of you. In the worst-case scenario, think of it as an experiment to see how your body feels. But don't be afraid of food.

CREATE YOUR OWN REALITY!

Remember: we create our own reality! Our thoughts have the power to bring themselves to life. Since feeling and showing gratitude and cultivating a feeling of love are such powerful tools why not use that power to create a better energy and acceptance for our own body?

Most of the time we talk about and focus on the things that we don't like about our bodies: flabby stomach, wrinkles, the wrong size of jeans, thin hair … the list goes on and on. Negative thoughts are limiting. We are programming "I can't" and "I don't" messages into low self-esteem and a negative body image. Now, understanding the science and the effect that focusing on the negative will have on your reality, you might think twice before going on a body-hate rant. Body image can change based on what you think and do every day. Listing positive things and things that you love about your body and your belly helps to reverse a negative self-image into a positive one. Whether you want to lose weight or eliminate bloating and digestive unease, choosing positive thoughts and supporting positive beliefs are a big part of the equation.

We become whatever we identify with. Your thoughts turn into your reality, whether you want it or not. We choose to identify with disease and become one with it. Maybe that's why some people get sick often while others don't get sick at all? It can also be the reason behind why some people have so much trouble losing weight: they have a picture of themselves as fat. What you visualize and focus on creates your body and everything that happens to you. Thoughts are food for the mind. We spend hours reading about nutrition and thinking about what to eat, but we rarely scrutinize our thoughts as closely as the restaurant menu. If you chose to feed your body with a clean, highly nutritional food, choose to feed your mind with positive and kind thoughts! You can use science and your own brain to change your body and improve your health.

Many people don't seem to get better even on a very strict diet and a hard-core supplement regimen — or if they do, their problems come right back. The reason is that your brain might still have an image of you being sick, bloated, and irregular, and that image is very powerful. Your brain will make sure that your body lives up to the internal belief. To make healing easier and permanent, the image of self has to be changed.

During my stay at the Hippocrates Institute in West Palm Beach, I was lucky enough to witness an amazing transformation of a third-stage breast-cancer patient. A beautiful young mother was at the Hippocrates Institute for three weeks to strengthen her body after struggling with cancer for 10 years and going through several courses of chemotherapy. In a group therapy session she sat in the circle, discussing her disease. The therapist didn't try to figure out her childhood patterns or inherited personality traits. He asked her one question: "Do you see yourself without cancer?"

The woman paused and then said, "No."

This realization that she couldn't even imagine her body without cancer made her break into tears. The wise therapist worked with her later in the session to help her create a new image: one without cancer. With her belief steadily increasing, the woman kept saying, "I am not my cancer. This cancer is not me."

Many women who have experienced bloating, IBS, or constipation for many years can't even imagine their lives without these accompanying partners.

Are you expecting to be bloated after certain foods? Do you firmly believe that you can't go to the bathroom without a laxative? Are you certain that a particular food will give you gas?

How deep are those beliefs, and how strong are those expectations? You might be creating a negative placebo effect for yourself (*nocebo*). If your self-image is fixed on a picture of you living with constipation, bloating, and gas, it can be very difficult to change things using diet alone.

These limiting beliefs and negative expectations need to be replaced with new empowering ones.

NATURAL TENDENCY FOR PROBLEM-SOLVING

Usually, if we are experiencing something unpleasant or painful, it becomes our only focus. When we encounter something negative, we pay extraordinary attention to it. Think about hearing a description of a stranger: "Joe is happy, confident, and funny. But he's cheap." Negative information like this can forecast a problem: if Joe is cheap, he may hoard, rather than share his resources with us.

A bloated stomach will get all the attention. A fear of feeling bad after a "bad" meal will hijack our mind. The discomfort of a constipated bowel can become the only focus—making us completely unproductive. Whatever we focus on grows.

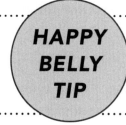

HAPPY BELLY TIP

Health gets better only when we focus on the desired state, instead of dread the negative present.

By complaining and suffering from what is, you gain no improvement. Improvement happens when you are clear on where you would like to be and how you would like to feel and start taking action to move closer to the desired state.

We should learn what is good for the body, the emotions, and the mind and identify with these thoughts. Then let us learn to stop identifying with those thoughts that are hurtful to us. The ancient sages and modern-day spirituality teachers, including Paul Brunton, say that those who have the ability to choose their thoughts at will have the ability to control their destiny. Those who accept only the right thoughts—who discriminatingly choose the thoughts that are conducive to the highest physical, emotional, and mental well-being—will perform the right actions at all times.

To change an existing pattern of negative expectations, regular meditation, visualization based on the wellness vision or positive imagery, and positive affirmations can work.

Here an easy exercise to get you started

For two weeks, try repeating positive affirmations about your digestion for two to three minutes a day. It is best if you can say them out loud, but if you feel too weird about it, say them in your head. You can also write them on your phone, a notepad, or the bathroom mirror to remind yourself. When saying the affirmation, pretend it's actually happening. Visualize it happening.

Here are some examples of positive affirmations that can help you with your belly:

- My digestion is strong and healthy.
- I digest the food well, assimilate all the nutrients, and eliminate all the waste.
- I have daily bowel movements.
- My intestines and colon are able to heal and be well again.
- My stomach is light, flat, and relaxed.
- I feel nourished and light after my meals.

Start small and build up to what feels natural. Keep affirmations positive, simple, and in the present tense. Doing this simple exercise will help you to reconnect with your body, to be proud of what it can do, and to feel grateful for everything that it allows you to do. Only humans have the power to find the positive even in challenging situations. Only we can control how we feel and what we focus our thoughts on. It is 100 percent your choice. The thoughts you have now are creating your tomorrow, and when you know that, you hold the tools to make all kinds of marvelous things happen.

....

chapter 20

TRACK YOUR PROGRESS AND LEARN FROM FAILURES

One of the goals that I would recommend, at least for the first four to six weeks, is to keep a daily food/symptom/emotions log.

This is an important step to get to know your body and your digestion. It will help to increase your awareness. You will start listening to your body and paying close attention to how it feels. Eventually, you will have a mental food map of foods that work for you and ones that don't. It will help you to know when and what to eat instead of feeling confused by all the nutrition advice out there.

You need to become a student of your body, listening intently, reviewing the material learned, and applying it to daily life. Let go of the notion that someone is going to solve your problems, make you feel better, or even know what works for your body. It is both empowering and scary, but it is true!

Maintaining a daily food and symptoms log is one of the fastest ways to learn about your digestion and the foods that work for it. It allows you to notice trends that you would not notice otherwise.

You will become more aware of your eating habits and stress and digestion connection. It does not have to be permanent; a food log is a temporary exercise that you use to increase mind/body understanding and connection.

In the beginning it might be a bit challenging. Many people start recording in the morning and then get busy and forget. It might happen to you for the first few days too. However, if you keep in mind that it is an important tool that will bring you knowledge that no expert can share with you, you will be motivated to find a few minutes a day to write your food choices and responses down. The sooner you would like to get rid of your symptoms, the more precise you should make your food log. Download a sample food/emotions/symptoms log at www. spinachandyoga.com/resources.

Everything should be noted: small meals, large meals, snacks, and drinks. Put down the time you ate, how you ate, your stress level, if you are stressed, and the way you felt after a meal. It literally cannot be too detailed. If you think it is relevant, put it down.

Among the things that you should track in your food log are your thoughts and expectations prior to the meals. Are you looking forward to something? Do you feel that you are eating the best food for you? Do you consider it nourishing to your body? Is there a fear of being bloated or unwell? Be mindful of those feelings and start noting them.

You will also use the log to document the changes in the way your digestive system functions. You will know what steps were the most effective and worked for your body. It is an essential tool that you must use daily to speed up the healing and to understand your body.

A daily log will also help you be more in touch with how you feel. To describe how you feel, you will start checking in with your body a lot more often: How I am feeling right now? How is my stomach feeling? What makes me feel my best? Describing it in words on paper can present a new perspective and give you a much deeper understanding.

A food log is not only for digestion. It will change your understanding of the integral functioning of all of the systems in the body. Your stomach and colon are not independent from all of the other organs of the body. What you eat affects how you feel, what emotions you experience, and how well you sleep, among other things. All bodily systems are interconnected in a very close and sensitive way. If things go wrong in the gut, it shows up everywhere. One of the benefits of keeping a daily food log is that you will gain awareness of certain trends that might be causing an issue in the first place.

I was amazed when, after a week of writing down my food, symptoms, and the things that occurred around food time, I noticed that I always ate in a rush. Breakfast was in a cab, rushing to see clients. Lunch was rushed in between appointments. Snacks were eaten while walking. Dinner was prepared in a rush because it was already late. Then I swallowed it in ten minutes because I was stressing out about not eating too late. The meals were healthy, but the way I was eating them was as unhealthy as it gets: no time to chew properly, to use all five senses, or to appreciate and savor the food. Only after looking at the weekly food log did I understand what caused my bloating and irregularity. It was not the food; it was my way of eating it.

One of my clients had a similar eye-opening experience. She used to suffer from high acidity, chocolate cravings, and skin hives. After tracking her foods, feelings, and digestion, she noticed that she was eating sour, fermented, hot and spicy things all day long! After taking those things out, she felt better within a few days.

The food log is a way to understand your body better, to be more aware of your symptoms, cravings, and eating patterns before jumping into any diet plans that might not address the root cause. When your eating patterns are unhealthy, just adding more veggies is not going to do the trick. You need to learn about your body to find your weakest point, your trigger situations or foods, and only then use this knowledge to set weekly goals. This is the smartest approach to getting back to your innate digestive balance.

First and foremost, you need to identify actions and things that aggravate digestion and lead to the unpleasant symptoms in the first place. Remember to download a fillable food/emotions/symptoms log at www.spinachandyoga.com/resources.

chapter 21
....

GOOD EATING HABITS

H abits are actions that we do on a regular basis often without even thinking. We discussed habits that hinder digestion earlier in the book, and now we will talk about habits that can foster a healthy digestion. This section covers *how* you eat rather than *what* to eat.

GENERAL HAPPY BELLY EATING HABITS

- Start your day with a glass of water with lime or lemon before anything else!

- Breathe and be present when you eat.

- Make eating a single-minded, sacred ceremony of nourishing your body.

- Eat slowly and mindfully.

- Eat portions that keep you satisfied but not stuffed.

- Allow the previous meal to fully digest before eating again. No grazing all day long.

- Refrain from eating two to three hours before bedtime.

- Follow simple food-combining rules.

- Drink plenty of warm water in small sips; avoid ice and cold water.

- No matter what you have on your plate, bless the food and let it be the best nourishment for your body.

- Find healthy ways to relieve stress such as meditation, movement, and relaxation.

- Practice yoga or stretching for improving digestive function and reducing stress.

- Limit your use of over-the-counter and prescription drugs.

- Limit caffeine and alcohol, which damage friendly bacteria.

Your habits around food will determine not only how well your digestion works but also your energy level, which is like money: there is never too much. The better your habits around food, the more energy-efficient your digestion will be and the more energy you will have to enjoy life, play, work, and change the world.

MINDFUL EATING 101

"When engaged in eating, the brain should be the servant of the stomach."

—AGATHA CHRISTIE

One of the most interesting writers and researchers on diet and health, Dr. Stanley Bass, who was 99 and still practicing in 2012, said, "Of all the subjects in existence, it is my considered opinion, after deep reflection, that what I am about to write is perhaps THE most important subject. A subject which can radically change a person's life in all of its aspects—physically, mentally, emotionally and spiritually: Attentive eating."[35]

He also, interestingly, said he believes that even if people refuse to change their diets to higher-quality foods and insist on remaining with their present conventional diet, they still will experience profound changes in all aspects of life by applying mindful eating to their habits.

Eating healthy portions and at the right time is not about self-control or exercising willpower. It is about listening to your body's signals and about eating mindfully. If you take time and commit to listening to your body, you won't have the problem of feeling stuffed or guilty after a meal. You will be able to join the ranks of people who can eat whatever they want without deprivation and without gaining weight. Sound like a dream? It's real, but learning to listen to your internal voice takes some practice, as does every other skill. The more you practice, the easier it becomes.

We taste something only while it's in our mouth. Once we swallow it, there's no more taste. It seems that, based on this fact, people who really enjoy the taste of sweets would slowly savor every bite and chew with full attention and focus. However, in reality, this isn't so. Often, we are so looking forward to the dessert that once it's in front of us, we eat it so fast that we can't even taste what we're devouring. Once nothing is left on the plate, we still feel hungry because we didn't get to enjoy the taste; our need for the taste of sweets hasn't been fulfilled. Seems like the most counterproductive situation, right? We wanted to enjoy the cake, but instead, we shoved it in so fast that the taste buds didn't even register the taste.

To change this unfortunate tendency and truly enjoy food, we have to be mindful at the table.

Mindful slow eating is good for you for several reasons

- It helps your digestion. Digestion starts in your mouth, and chewing food will significantly reduce the workload for your stomach.

- It will help you lose unhealthy weight. By eating more slowly, you will fill up with less food and consume fewer calories. It takes about 20 minutes for our brains to register that we're full. If we eat fast, we can continue eating past the point where we're full. If we eat slowly, we have time to realize we're full and stop in time.

- It can reduce your stress level. Consciously slowing down and bringing awareness into any process will help reduce stress. It can become your time for mindfulness meditation or exercise. Try to be completely present in your body while consuming food.

- You will enjoy food more and have fewer cravings. Often we crave something for days but as soon as we get it, we gobble it down in a second without actually tasting the food. There is no feeling of satisfaction, and the cravings soon return. Savoring each piece and mentally acknowledging a food's taste will allow your brain to register a pleasant moment and will make you feel satisfied.

Turn on the Senses

If you look back at some of your most memorable meals, you'll find that your most enjoyable moments at the table have been when most of your senses were engaged. You got to see, smell, touch, taste, and listen.

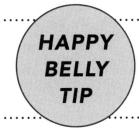

HAPPY BELLY TIP To turn food into a sensual, fulfilling experience, you need to learn to turn on all the senses.

Unfortunately, turning all the senses on is impossible when you are in a rush. Senses require time; they won't fully turn on until you slow down. Using all your senses and slowing down is what makes mindful eating different from mindless munching.

Try these tips to master mindful eating:

- Start by taking a few deep breaths before eating. It will help you to shift out of an in-a-rush frame of mind and into a more peaceful state of mind. Breathe!

- Eat as you would at a super fancy restaurant. Appreciate the smell, presentation, and taste. Take mindful bites and put your spoon/fork down while you chew, instead of filling up the utensil for the next one. Take time to absorb the colors, smell, and flavors of the food. Mentally or aloud, use three to five adjectives to describe what's on your plate.

- Try to avoid multitasking and focus solely on the taste of the food. When you talk, talk; when you chew, don't talk.

- Make at least one meal a day a self-sufficient event. Whether you are with your friends, family, or alone, sit at the table, use a plate and utensils (even if you bought a take-out-deli sandwich).

- Chew each bite. Sometimes I notice people mindlessly putting spoonful after spoonful in their mouth and swallowing almost without chewing. The plate won't disappear in five minutes after you start eating, so slow down and enjoy your meal. A good strategy is to put the utensils down in between each bite and focus on experiencing the taste and flavor. (If you are afraid that your food will get cold, use stoneware, warm up plates in the oven before serving, or serve smaller portions and go for seconds.)

- Listen to your body's feedback after the meal or snack. How does it feel in your stomach? What emotions or thoughts come up before and after your meal? No judgments here, just awareness.

Mindful eating is a skill that takes practice before it becomes a habit. Commit to it daily and take it one little step at a time. The more you practice, the better you will feel, and the easier it will become.

WHEN YOU EAT MATTERS

The best time for us to eat is when our body is ready to digest food. It means you will digest your best when you are in a relaxed state and not tired. While having lunch as the main meal would be optimal for digestion, leaving your body plenty of time to deal with a complex meal, this might not be the best option if you have a busy 9–5 job. Taking an hour to eat and then 30 minutes to rest after a big meal might be too big of a luxury during a workday. However, if you can make it happen, by all means do it!

I find that if I have a busy day, I feel better leaving my main meal for later when I feel more relaxed and settled. When busy and stressed, go for easy-to-digest simple meals with just a few ingredients.

During the weekend or during celebrations, it might be better to have the biggest meal earlier in the day. Our body prepares to rest in the evening and having a heavy meal at 9 p.m. will interfere with this natural cycle. The quality of sleep and digestion will suffer as a result. If you don't have a choice and the social event is scheduled for later in the evening, eat something beforehand and focus on socializing at the group dinner. I do it all the time, since a weekend 9 p.m. dinner in New York City is considered normal. In the beginning, my boyfriend would find it awkward that I ate before going to the restaurant, but he got used to it.

You choose your priorities and the behaviors that support your priorities. If a late dinner interferes with your digestion the next day, make arrangements to eat earlier. Do it with a smile, without complaining, and still have fun when you get to the social event. In the end, the whole point of getting together is to socialize, and food is just a medium. If you don't make a big deal out of a late dinner and don't make people feel guilty for having unhealthy habits, no one will care that you are not eating or just having a soup.

Allow your previous meal to fully digest before eating again. Do not graze all day long. Make sure that you wait at least three to four hours after a regular meal. A meal of fruit or vegetables will require less time to digest. If you have grains, protein, and vegetables in one meal, definitely wait four hours before eating again. Be kind to your digestive system and let it deal with one meal at a time.

Refrain from eating two to three hours before bedtime so you get a good night of sleep and don't force your digestion to work when it is not meant to.

HOW MUCH

Overeating hurts digestion, period. No matter what you eat too much of, it is an unhealthy behavior. Yogic texts from the ancient times recommend eating no more than 3/4 the size of the stomach. Modern nutritionists usually recommend not eating more than you can put into two, open, cupped hands.

Without measuring stomach size or putting your food in your hands, you can determine if you eat appropriate portions by how you feel after your meals. We only become aware of parts of our body if there is a problem. If you become aware of your stomach after your meals, you've probably eaten too much.

Based on the previous experience, you will be able to determine what is a good portion for you. One of the kindest things you can do for your digestive system is not to overload it.

UNDERSTAND YOUR DIGESTIVE INDICATORS

Only eat when you are hungry! We often eat out of habit rather than need. Before you eat, score your hunger on a scale of 1–10. Anything over six or seven and you probably need some nourishment; anything less, go and find something more interesting to do to distract you from your craving. Alternatively, go and drink something like water or a fruit tea, as we often mistake dehydration for hunger.

The more you practice rating your hunger before meals, the easier it will become. Soon you will be able to differentiate between emotional, physical, and mental hunger, as well as hunger versus fullness. Awareness of your body is your best teacher. Listen to it.

FOOD COMBINING

Food combination theories can be quite complicated to understand, and almost impossible to remember right away. However, there is one key rule that will save you a lot of memorizing: simplicity. The fewer ingredients, the fewer different enzymes you need to digest food and the less likely the food will get stuck in your body, fermenting and depleting your energy levels. The longer the food ferments in your stomach, the more likely you will feel bloated, sluggish, and heavy. Simple meals are easier because they require fewer resources to break down and turn into nutrients.

Another rule is keeping portions manageable. If you know that you will be eating a complicated meal consisting of hard-to-digest products, keep the amount small. It is easier to deal with a small problem than a large one.

Here are the top 10 rules of food combining (FC) that I use and that you might find interesting to experiment with.

1. **The simpler the meal, the easier it will be to digest.** Keep the ingredients few but make them count.

2. **Dairy should not be combined with pretty much anything besides greens and nonstarchy vegetables.** Baked goat cheese on veggies or salads is okay, but no pizza, cream-based pasta sauces, or dairy-based chowders. When it comes to yogurt, add vanilla bean or honey and cinnamon, but no jams or fruits.

3. **Fruit should not be combined with anything because it is digested a lot faster than most other things.** It is best to eat fruit at least 20 minutes before anything else. Fruits require a lot less time to digest, but if there is already something in your stomach, they will sit there and ferment, which will give you an uncomfortable bloated feeling. Fruit with grains, fruit with eggs, fruit with nuts, and fruit after a meal are among the infamous no-nos. The only exception is dried fruit boiled together with grains, as in oatmeal or an occasional treat with homemade cookies or muffins baked with berries or dried fruit.

4. **Have one concentrated protein per meal.** This one is pretty simple: no fish and chicken, meat and shrimp, eggs and milk, cheese and beans on one plate. A meal of combined proteins will take 10–12 hours to digest if you have a strong digestion. Why would you want to voluntarily sign up for 12 hours of nonstop work?

5. **If you have carbs and animal protein in one meal, try to eat them sequentially.** Eat carbs first and protein last. The reasoning behind it can be found in Dr. Stanley Bass's sequential eating theory. In his article "Ideal Health through Sequential Eating,"[36] Dr. Bass describes how different foods eaten in a light-to-heavy sequence are digested in layers and leave the stomach in sequences. If you eat a meal of fruit, followed by a salad, followed by baked squash, and finish with eggs, fruit will leave the stomach first—after 30 minutes. Then the second layer (tossed salad) will move into its place, leaving the stomach in about 30 to 40 minutes. This is followed by the third layer (squash), which then moves down and will be the next to leave the stomach. As the meal progresses, you should eat foods that

FOOD TRANSIT TIMES

Water	0–15 minutes
Juice	15–30 minutes
Fruit	30–60 minutes
Melons	30–60 minutes
Sprouts	60 minutes
Wheatgrass Juice	60–90 minutes
Most Vegetables	1–2 hours
Grains and Beans	1–2 hours
Dense Vegetable Protein	2–3 hours
Meat and Fish	3–4 hours +
Shellfish	8 hours +
Any Improperly Combined Meal	8 hours

SERVING SIZE

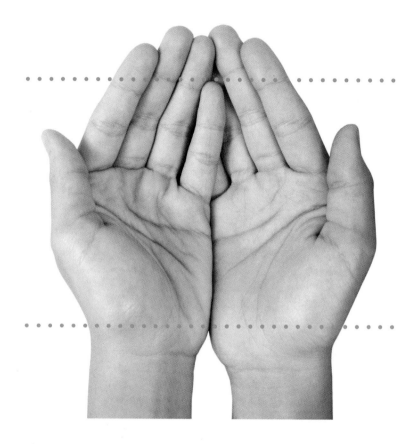

Overeating hurts digestion, period. Overeating is unhealthy, no matter what you are consuming. Yogic texts from the ancient times recommend eating an amount no more than 3/4 the size of the stomach. Modern nutritionists usually recommend not eating more than you can put into two, open, cupped hands.

FOOD COMBINING

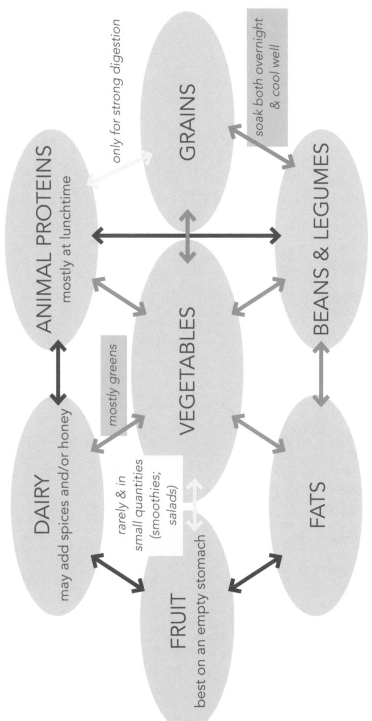

Good combinations

Okay for occasional use

Keep these combinations to a minimum

DAIRY
may add spices and/or honey

ANIMAL PROTEINS
mostly at lunchtime

GRAINS

BEANS & LEGUMES

VEGETABLES

FATS

FRUIT
best on an empty stomach

only for strong digestion

soak both overnight & cool well

mostly greens

rarely & in small quantities (smoothies; salads)

HAPPY BELLY GREEN SOUP RECIPE

This soup is easy to digest and supergood for your body. It can be an accompaniment to breakfast, lunch, or dinner. I love to have it in all seasons, just switching up seasonal veggies and spices. Once you get the hang of the process, you will be able to create your favorite variations. Make it thinner or thicker, depending on your preference. Feel free to add hemp seeds, avocado, almond, or coconut milk for a richer variation. It is fast, simple, and belly-friendly! Serve it with a sprouted toast or eggs, quinoa, or a side of wild salmon. All variations are possible; trust your taste buds!

INGREDIENTS:

serves 4

- 1 tbsp olive oil or ghee
- 1 inch fresh ginger, peeled, and chopped
- 1 lb fresh spinach leaves (any leafy greens: arugula, kale, watercress, mash)
- 4 cups water or nondairy milk
- Sea salt, fresh lime juice, and pepper to taste
- Optional: hemp seeds

- 2 cloves garlic, chopped (kills bad bacteria)
- 4 cups fresh zucchini (or broccoli, cauliflower, or any seasonal vegetable)
- A handful of fresh cilantro, roughly chopped
- 2 tsp curry powder or dosha-specific spice mix (order at Banyan Botanicals)
- To garnish: Flax seed crackers , quinoa salad, or good-quality whole grain bread

1. Heat the ghee or olive oil in a large pot over medium heat. Add garlic and chopped ginger, stirring until translucent. Add the curry powder or your dosha mix, and salt to taste. Cook for 1 minute. Add the zucchini and stir to mix well. Add enough water to cover the zucchini; bring to a boil and simmer for 10 minutes, or until the zucchini is just tender.

2. Using a blender or food processor, puree the zucchini mixture with spinach, cilantro, water or nondairy milk, and hemp seeds. Add more hot water if the soup is too thick. Transfer back to the pot and bring to a simmer and season with black pepper and a squeeze of lime juice.

3. Serve over crumbled flax seed crackers or top with quinoa salad.

CLASSIC KITCHARI

INGREDIENTS

3-4 servings

- 1 cup split yellow mung beans (soaked overnight)
- ½ tsp ghee or coconut oil
- 1 tsp each: black mustard seeds, cumin, and turmeric powder
- 1 pinch hing (asafetida)
- ½ tsp salt (rock salt is best)
- ½ lime

- 1 cup long grain white or brown basmati rice (can use quinoa too)
- 1 tbsp fresh ginger root
- ½ tsp each: coriander powder, fennel, and fenugreek seeds
- 7–10 cups water
- 1 small handful fresh, chopped, cilantro leaves

Optional: beets, kale, zucchini, carrots, cauliflower, green beans, or any other vegetable you like

WHAT TO DO

1. Soak beans and grains overnight (or at least for a few hours). Rinse well.
2. Heat ghee and mustard seeds in a large saucepan on medium heat until seeds begin to pop. Add remaining spices and cook briefly.
3. Add the water before the spices burn.
4. Add grains, dal, and salt. Bring to a boil and cook for 10 minutes.
5. Add hard vegetables, such as beets and carrots, cover and simmer until dal, veggies, and rice/quinoa are soft, approx 30 mins. Add additional water as necessary.
6. Add softer vegetables and greens 5 minutes before grains and lentils are fully cooked.
7. Add the cilantro leaves and lime juice right before serving.

VARIATIONS

- Coconut Raisin Breakfast Goodness: 1/2 tsp cardamon, cinnamon, a handful of raisins, and 2–3 tbs coconut flakes.
- Mediterranean Adventure: 1/4 cup fresh dill, juice from 1/2 a lemon. Sea salt and pepper to taste.   *(continued on next page)*

VARIATIONS CONT'D.

- Chai Breakfast Bowl: add chai masala powder or 1/4 tsp cardamom powder, 3 cloves, 1 stick cinnamon, 1 tsp ginger powder, and a dash of black pepper. Top with 2-3 chopped dates.
- Pesto: Boil without ghee and before serving add your favorite vegan pesto sauce. Serve with lemon and black pepper.
- Seaside Bowl: Cook with sesame oil, add 1 tsp ginger powder and hijiki seaweed when cooking. After cooking, add miso paste to taste. Sprinkle with flakes of seaweed dulse or crumbled nori and sesame seeds.

KIND CURRIED CAULIFLOWER SOUP

INGREDIENTS:

yields 4-5 cups

- 1 large head cauliflower, chopped
- 1 large handful of arugula leaves
- ¼ inch fresh ginger
- 4 cups water
- 1 tsp turmeric powder
- 3 tbsp toasted sesame seeds
- salt and pepper to taste

- 1 tbsp ghee (substitute sesame seeds or olive oil for a vegan version)
- 2 cloves garlic, minced
- 2 tsp curry powder
- 3 tbsp hemp seeds
- To garnish: flax seed crackers

1. Heat the ghee in a large pot over medium heat. Add garlic and chopped ginger, stirring until translucent. Add the curry powders, turmeric, and salt to taste. Cook for 1 minute. Add the cauliflower and stir to mix well. Add enough water to cover the cauliflower; bring to a boil and simmer for 10 minutes, or until the cauliflower is just tender.

2. Using a blender or food processor, puree the cauliflower mixture with hemp seeds and toasted sesame seeds. Add more hot water if the soup is too thick. Transfer back to the pot, bring to a simmer, and season with black pepper. Add chopped arugula and mix.

3. Serve over crumbled flax seed crackers.

EASY VS. HARD-TO-DIGEST FOODS

EASY	HARD
Most cooked veggies: carrot, celery, okra, sweet potatoes, zucchini	Cheese: hard and soft. Old, molded, ripened cheeses are harder.
Cooked apples, pears	All cabbage family: cabbage, cauliflower, broccoli, brussels sprouts
Berries, oranges, peaches, grapefruit, kiwi, watermelon, lime, lemon, banana	Dry nuts: hazelnuts, brazil nuts, cashews, macadamias, peanuts, pecans, pistachios, walnuts
Greens: arugula, baby greens, watercress, endive	Red meat: beef, pork, rabbit
Most vegetables: carrots, kale, green beans, sweet potatoes, yellow onion, garlic, horseradish, zucchini, butternut squash, okra	Most beans (larger ones are harder): adzuki, black beans, chickpeas, cannellini, lentils, black eyed peas, kidney beans, fava beans, lima, split peas
Egg whites	Cheese (older, ripened, molded ones are harder): feta, mozzarella, blue cheese, parmesan
Sunflower seeds	Heavy grains: Wheat, brown and wild rice
Light grains: Rice, quinoa, oats, spelt, barley	Sweets: baked goods, candy, chocolate
Mung beans, sweet peas	Heavy fats: animal fat, coconut milk, heavy cream
Goat milk	Corn and all corn products
Avocado	Egg yolk
Coconut water	Soy products: soy beans, tofu, soy cheeses
Fish	Baked and bread products: yeasted bread, wheat bread, rye bread, seitan (wheat meat)
Spices: fennel, black pepper, cayenne, cinnamon, cumin, cloves, cilantro, caraway seeds, anise, basil, mint, paprika	Diary products: milk
Some fermented products: miso, apple cider vinegar	Some vegetables: Pumpkin, mushrooms, parsnip, tomato
Simple vegetable soups, porridges, liquid-based monomeals such as kitchari, blended room-temperature soups and smoothies made with spices such as ginger and cardamom	Packaged and processed products. Leftovers, frozen food, and stale food

HEALING STORIES

Sue Ellen ....

Most of my adult life I'd lived what would be considered a "healthy noncouch potato life style." But in April 2006, I was diagnosed with pernicious anemia, which means that my body would not process the essential vitamin B12, along with full-blown erosive gastritis, and psoriasis. To top it off, my blood sugar levels were soaring.

I had experienced cramping, bloating, poorly formed stool, and significant stomach and bowel distress. I could never be far from the bathroom.

I decided that I was not going to live the rest of my life taking as many prescription meds as were required to continue my normal day-to-day activities without experimenting to see if there was a more natural way, a way that might actually cure the disease rather than just lessen its symptoms.

I did some research on my own and decided to put myself on an elimination diet for six weeks with no gluten, no sweeteners of any kind, and no dairy. A couple of weeks into the diet, I lost ten pounds and experienced a lessening in bloating. My bowel movements, which had been so problematic without the meds, were "normal" and have remained so. As I approached the six-week mark, the mildly annoying chronic aches across my back were gone. Frequent headaches—gone. Aching joints—gone. The psoriasis? Even more improvement. And I'd lost another ten pounds.

Armed with my discoveries, I decided to explore further my growing conviction of two basic truths: 1) the body wants to heal itself, and 2) we have a lot of control over that. I needed a guide to steer my journey.

Nadya's gentle guidance and keen ability to listen provided me with several suggested tools that I immediately incorporated and continue to practice:

- pay attention to how I feel more than numbers on lab reports or weight;
- warm water with fresh lime juice to start my day;
- no caffeine on an empty stomach;
- add more soft, warm, and nourishing foods;
- only one protein at a meal;
- eat fresh fruit only on an empty stomach and at least thirty minutes before other foods.

Ayurveda, fundamentally, is the art of listening to one's body, noticing subtle responses to food and food combinations, and, for me, establishing a routine, which in turn becomes an anchor. This framework of self-care expands naturally to include mood, response to stress, and even crisis management.

Without hesitation, I can say I have never felt better in my adult life. I am excited about increasing my knowledge and practice of self-care.

My two theories are proving true: the body wants to heal itself, and I have everything to say about whether or not that will happen through the many daily choices I make. I anticipate my retirement years will be filled with great, creative cooking adventures, and fortified with the daily practices that anchor me: morning hygiene rituals, yoga, meditation, and prayer.

I am learning to think of self-care not as a chore, or a selfish use of time, but as a precious gift to myself, which then becomes a gift to others.

Jasmine S. Glass

Sluggish digestion has caused many issues for me. Since childhood, I could not handle dairy or meat, but I kept eating those foods. During that time, I dealt with severe constipation. At age 6, I suffered from an impacted bowel. Since I couldn't pass anything, I also could not eat. Many conventional MDs gave me the typical advice of consuming more fiber, drinking more water, and getting more exercise. These answers were very frustrating, as I was a very healthy athlete at the time. I became a vegetarian, went vegan, and then decided not to eat at all. I developed cystic acne. I became extremely irritable, fell into depression, and my overall personality changed.

The thought of eating out gave me a tremendous amount of anxiety. I was afraid to put myself out in the world. I felt too ugly, I felt too weird and anxiety-ridden. I closed myself off and made myself feel bad about it.

Soon I realized that I had to search for answers outside Western medicine. I laid off over-the-counter quick fixes and began to search for my answers in the produce section. Ayurveda has played a big role. Discovering ayurveda felt as if I had hit a jackpot. The mind-body connection spoke to me the most. Not only did I have explanations for my physical ailments but also reasons why my mental and emotional mentalities changed. The depression, the anxiety, the irritability was more than just a case of lack of confidence or low self-esteem.

I learned about herbs, teas, and detoxification. Hot lemon water, burdock root, and dandelion all have taken the place of harsh chemicals for my skin ailments and headaches. I've adopted many habits: checking my tongue, fingernails, and poop to monitor my health.

I feel absolutely amazing. My skin is bright and glowing. It doesn't feel hot or inflamed. My aches and pains are eradicated, and my poop is regular and satisfactory. I make much more effort and take much more initiative to be the healthiest I can be.

The most wonderful thing I've learned about my body is the fact that it has the complete ability to heal itself if I give it the right resources: healthy foods, antioxidants, healthy fats, sunlight, water, herbs, exercise, a positive attitude, an active spiritual life. I have learned that everything about the human body is linked or connected. A pain in my back could be caused by a wheat sensitivity that has triggered inflammation in my body. Who knew that a sandwich could cause back pain?

If you are not happy with your current state, don't give up. Experiment and find your answers. At the age of 19, I can say that ayurveda has drastically saved my social life, helped me spiritually and emotionally, kept my physical body in shape and so on and so forth. However, I did not get to this point without using myself as a human guinea pig. Everyone's body is different and the only way you will improve your body is to do your own research and experiment with yourself. Good health is not a destination; it is a journey.

For more personal stories and inspiration, go to www.spinachandyoga.com/healingstories

HAPPY BELLY MEAL PLAN

This seven-day meal plan is designed by Dana James and Nadya Andreeva to nourish your body without overloading digestion. All recipes are well-combined, anti-inflammatory, nutrient rich, gluten-, dairy-, soy-, and sugar-free. All the recipes can be found at www.spinachandyoga.com/recipes.

DAY	BREAKFAST	SNACK (only if hungry)	LUNCH (biggest meal if possible)	SNACK (only if hungry)	DINNER (light and simple)
DAY 1	Warm green soup and 2 eggs (only egg whites if high Pitta)	Raspberries	Home-made lentil soup with veggies and 1/2 avocado	Mint tea with four soaked prunes	Minestrone soup with flax seed crackers or sprouted gluten-free bread
DAY 2	Quinoa with veggies	Chai latte with almond milk	Black bean burgers with avocado sauce and roasted roots	Fennel tea; pear	Roasted fennel and butternut squash soup
DAY 3	Hemp Smoothie	Applesauce with spices	Mash salad with poached salmon	Coriander tea; Avocado sprinkled with lime juice and pepper	Spaghetti squash casserole with sautéed spinach

DAY 4	Chia pudding	1/2 grapefruit	Kitchari and sautéed greens (can have salad if no tendency to bloat and it is warm outside)	Chamomile tea; handful of pumpkin seeds	Mung bean soup and roasted or sautéed seasonal vegetables
DAY 5	Quinoa or amaranth with dried fruits and almonds	Acai chai	Seaweed salad with daikon and sesame seeds. Yellow lentil soup	Pumpkin pie or Summer Joy smoothie	Crockpot vegetable stew and 1/2 avocado. Sprinkle with cilantro
DAY 6	Stewed apple with spices and 10 soaked almonds	Handful of sunflower seeds and tea	Zucchini pasta and wild salmon	Herbal tea; Chia seed pudding	Omelet with veggies and green soup
DAY 7	Poached eggs over sautéed greens	Pear	Black beans and quinoa (can substitute for any other grain) over massaged avocado kale	Herbal tea; zucchini hummus with 1/4 avocado	Roasted asparagus and grilled white fish

SHOPPING LIST AND NOTES

AYURVEDIC PLATES

Images created by Caroline Thaw

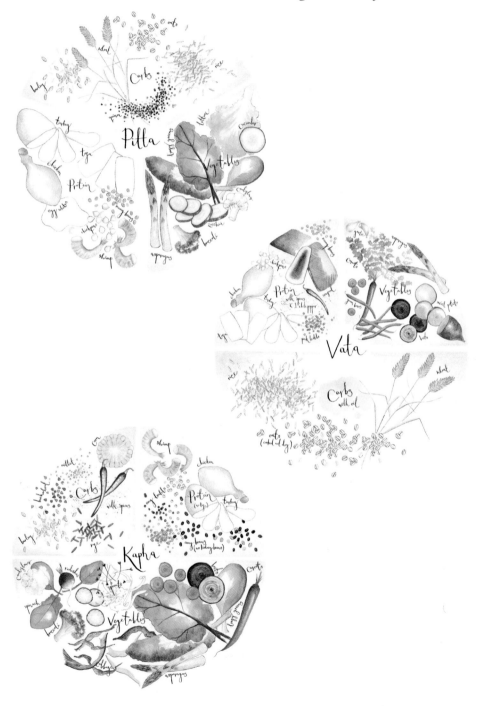

require a longer time for processing in the stomach. According to Dr. Bass, the most watery, least dense foods should be eaten first, and the most concentrated or dense foods should be eaten last. Watery foods, such as fresh fruits and leafy salads, are digested rapidly, leaving the stomach quickly and making room for the more concentrated foods. This prevents fermentation and bloating which could occur if everything is mixed and chewed together and gets into the stomach in one mass. Considering that, at the age of 99, Dr. Bass still has plenty of energy to do research, write, and treat clients, there might be something to his theory. I certainly notice a big difference. For me, sequential eating has become a habit.

6. **Drink a little bit of warm water or herbal tea before a meal,** a little bit during, and nothing after for at least 30 minutes after. It prevents gastric juices from diluting and allows for better digestion.

7. **Soak all nuts overnight.** It makes them less dry and easier to break down. They become a lot less heavy. Add nuts to vegetable dishes and curries, but do not overdo them as dry snacks, especially with dried fruit, because they are oily, dense, and heavy.

8. **Always add greens when having fats with proteins or starches.** When fats are eaten with green vegetables, the inhibiting effect of fats on gastric secretion is counteracted and digestion proceeds quite normally. Many vitamins and minerals absorb better with the presence of fat. Try lentils with avocado and sautéed kale or baked sweet potato with ghee and a side of arugula salad.

9. **Let your body rest at least once per week by eating monomeals.** We will discuss this in detail later in the book.

10. **When in doubt about a certain food combination, try to pay attention to your body's feedback.** Your body knows better than any nutritionist. Sometimes our bodies are so accustomed to a certain combination that we can digest it quite well even though it might not fit by the book. It depends on your cultural traditions and the strength of digestion.

My clients often ask me: how strictly should you follow food combination rules?

Below is my honest answer. This approach works well for me and should be a good starting point for you if you are just experimenting with FC.

I follow FC more strictly when I am busy or under stressful circumstances to help my body deal with the stress better. In general, I would say I follow it 80 percent of time, and 20 percent of the time I am pretty relaxed about the rules.

When sick or tired, I follow food combining more strictly to help my body preserve energy for housekeeping and healing. When healthy and rested, I relax the rules since I know that my body can afford to expend more energy on digestion without making me feel tired.

Avoid difficult combinations at night or at least three to four hours before sleep. Soups, cooked vegetables, and salads with light dressings and sometimes an egg-white omelet are my go-to in the evening.

When I do combine hard-to-digest foods such as carbs and proteins and fats in one meal, I eat smaller quantities, focus on checking in with my stomach throughout the meal, eat the densest food (protein) last, and wait at least four to five hours before the next meal.

CHANGING HABITS THE LOVING WAY

No herbs, supplements, or prescriptions can overcome the effects of poor eating habits.

Habit formation is the process by which new behaviors become automatic. If you instinctively reach for a sweet after lunch or dinner, you have a habit. In the same way, if you drink a glass of warm water with lime first thing in the morning, you build a habit. According to *Psychology Today* old habits are hard to break, and new habits are hard to form. That's because the behavioral patterns we repeat most often are literally etched in our neural pathways. The good news is that through repetition, it's possible to form new habits.

Mark Twain reportedly said about habits, "Quitting smoking is the easiest thing in the world. I know because I've done it thousands of times."

Consciousness, awareness, paying attention without judgment— these are all cognitive tools that help high achievers stick to their goals. It is not the same as using force or willpower when adopting a new habit. When people make a resolution to stop eating a certain food (let's say gluten) or to start doing a regular self-care practice (let's say mindful breathing), 88 percent of them will fail, according to a survey conducted by the British psychologist Richard Wiseman.[37] We resist forceful change, we don't like to rely on willpower, and motivation does not always help.

In my work with women, I notice that they do better if they are inspired, not forced or motivated. Creating a change from a place that feels comfortable, loving, exciting, and beautiful comes easier than a change that comes from limitation, an attempt to "fix" something broken, or to push through. Your life should not feel tense, controlled, and stressful if you are adopting a new way of eating and a new way of caring for your body and digestion in particular. The change will be easier if you still enjoy your life on a daily basis and have a beautiful, exciting vision that keeps you inspired to take action every single day. This is why coming back to your wellness vision on a regular basis in the beginning has one of the most powerful effects on change.

Evaluating Where You Are with Your Habits

Our emotions, thoughts, and behavioral patterns affect our physical body. It is important to take an honest look at where you stand now before jumping into behavior change.

Start by taking a nonjudgmental look at the following questions.

- What and how do you think about your meals? Is there a sense of stress, confusion, feeling overwhelmed, restriction, control, gracefulness, pleasure, relaxation, or playfulness?

- What do you eat on a daily basis? Are your meals nourishing and nutrient-dense?

- How often do you snack? How often do you overeat? Do you binge?

- What kind of eater are you? If you were to look at yourself eating, what would you say? Are you a fast, rushed, stressed eater? Or are you slow and graceful? Do you savor and enjoy your food or angrily shove the food into your mouth, spoonful after spoonful as if you were on a mission to get the food in as quickly as possible?

- What does your food look like? Is it pretty and colorful or messy and dull looking?

- What foods are your staples? How would you describe those staple foods in terms of their qualities (e.g., greens: light, bright, vital, anti-inflammatory; chocolate: hot, sharp, acidic, stimulating)? We take in the qualities of the food and over time, our body and personality will portray more of those qualities.

SMART GOALS

Wellness goals are what help you to get from your present state to your ideal wellness state. Goals rarely fail because of a lack of commitment or enthusiasm. They die for lack of a compelling vision with a plan designed to achieve it. With a vision, you imagine an outcome that you then make come to life through the goals you set. A goal that is not tied to some kind of vision will often just "float out there" with a vague sense of importance. To create a clear picture of your ideal self and your ideal digestion, write out answers to all the questions in the chapter on wellness vision (page 131) before jumping to goals.

Once you know where you would like to move, it's time to create SMART goals. You will be able to create smart goals using your own knowledge, intuition, and the strategies outlined in this book. Now we are just covering goal-setting theory.

One of the most important steps in creating a healthier you is setting goals in a way that is empowering and exciting. These goals should be based on where you want to be in the future, on the best ideal self that you are thriving to become.

SMART is an acronym for *specific, measurable, actionable, realistic,* and *timely.* People who use SMART goals are more likely to succeed in their quest for better health, healthy weight, and a sense of joy and fulfillment in daily life. By crafting SMART goals, you will obtain clear, concise feedback regarding your progress. Here are some tips for turning a general goal in a SMART goal.

Pick only three goals to begin with. Pick well! If you are working with a nutritionist, integrative doctor, or gastroenterologist, try not to commit to too many changes to prevent the process from being overwhelming. Think what three changes would be the most beneficial but the least stressful. As you may recall, stressing out will just make things worse.

If you are doing it on your own, be very honest with yourself about your current behaviors and diet and choose based on what would help you move closer to the wellness vision you want to bring into reality.

Below is an example of a thought process behind building a goal. For more examples and to download a goal-setting tool, go to www.spinachandyoga.com/resources.

General goal: Reduce bloating and have a flat stomach.

Turning the goal SMART

- **Specific**—Saying that you want to reduce bloating in order to have a flat stomach is great but not very specific.

Instead, decide exactly what you would like to do. After analyzing your habits, see if you can pinpoint a behavior that creates bloating in the first place and then choose to substitute it with a behavior that would support digestion. For example, your goal is to strive to stop eating when 80 percent full. Another goal that would help reduce bloating would be to follow food-combining rules. The more specific the better!

- **Measurable**—Give your goal a number so you can measure success and follow through. Let's say you want to stop eating junk food that makes you bloated, so you can make "five days out of seven with no junk food" your goal. If your goal is to do an elimination diet and determine if food sensitivity is causing bloating, you could say, "Find 10 gluten- and dairy-free recipes that I love and buy groceries to make them." Five handfuls of greens per day is measurable; "a lot of greens" is not!

- **Action-oriented**—The goals should be based on behaviors that result in change. Our goal of finding 10 recipes fits well. However, the second goal—our plan to stay away from junk food five days out of seven—is not actionable. It does not specify what you are going to eat instead of junk food! So to make it actionable, it would be better to state it this way: "I will eat unprocessed balanced meals with protein, greens, starchy vegetables, and healthy fats five days a week."

- **Realistic**—Many people fail to reach their goals because they set their standards too high. A healthy challenge is motivating; unrealistic goals are demotivating. Don't set yourself up for a failure! Saying that you will never again eat cookies is not realistic; saying that you will have nutrient-dense vegetables and protein at least two times per day is more realistic.

- **Time-bound**—Having a deadline will move you ahead more rapidly, so establish some for each goal. Include both short- and long-term goals. Reevaluate your goals on a weekly basis to assess what has worked or what interventions you need to help yourself along. Remember, it takes three to six months for new habits to become permanent and to begin to see noticeable changes. Give yourself time.

Examples of SMART goals

- I will drink warm water with lime/lemon first thing in the morning before having breakfast, every day for two weeks, before reevaluating my goal.

- I will do an elimination diet with no gluten or dairy for two weeks, focusing on vegetables, healthy protein, and fruits and then reevaluate my goals.

- I will do one minute of slow, deep breathing through the nose before lunch and dinner to relax, focus on how I want to feel at the end of the meal, and be more mindful. I will do it for seven days before reevaluating my goal.

- I will take three minutes after breakfast to do a visualization of how I want my stomach to work and what I want it to look like. I will use my wellness vision for inspiration. I will do it Monday, Wednesday, and Friday this week.

When choosing your goals, choose based on your desired outcome and be honest about what you are willing and not willing to do. Act from the place where you are now and don't try to completely overhaul your diet and lifestyle in one week.

At the end of every week, evaluate your success and lessons. What came easily, what stressed you out, what can you learn and use for the future? Learning is the most important take-away from the weekly goal review. Without it, you might face an issue week in, week out and never come up with a solution. Thinking back about your progress, celebrating it, and learning from failures is a key to the smart approach to wellness.

It is important to choose realistic goals that you can achieve and that will help to build self-trust and confidence. I really like the way Leo Babauta, the founder of Zen Habits, and a master of changing habits, writes about self-trust during the process of habit change in his *Little Contentment* book:

> Your relationship with yourself is like your relationship with anyone else. If you have a friend who is constantly late and breaking his word, not showing up when he says he will, eventually you'll stop trusting that friend. It's like that with your self too. It's hard to like someone you don't trust, and it's hard to like yourself if you don't trust yourself. So work on this trust with yourself. Increase it slowly, and eventually you'll trust yourself to be awesome.[38]

To increase self-trust, set realistic goals that are challenging but achievable. I can't tell you enough how important it is to create realistic, clear goals. This step will determine whether you move forward or stay stuck.

Writing your goal on paper and creating a plan around it to achieve it is very powerful. To make it even more powerful, exchange your goals with a friend.

What If Your Bad Eating Habits Are Very Sticky?

You are not alone. We all have a hard time changing habits and giving up habits that are not doing us any good. It is not easy to say no to the old comforting habit of having snacks all day at the computer, while you work on projects that are boring you out of your mind. It is hard to give up the dessert after dinner that you look forward to every day. Eating fast while checking e-mails could be a habit that keeps you "productive" and multitasking in the fast-paced world. How can you slow down? Emotional eating is never easy to control. Otherwise, everybody would control it. All bad habits are very sticky.

When you gain awareness of the habits that are hurting your digestion and your health, don't start a war against them. First, ask why they are there. Then, slowly find a way to fulfill the need that they are meeting with other habits that are kinder to your belly.

Awareness of your thoughts and emotions will come in very handy here. It is not a skill that we are usually taught, but it is a great skill to learn at any point of your life if you are serious about changing old habits that might be hurting your body. You must be very alert when working with old patterns.

Dr. Stanley Bass encourages you not to start a fight with temptation. Instead, he encourages you to shift your awareness to a positive goal and the reason that you started your journey to begin with. The very moment you realize that an undesirable craving/old habit has entered your consciousness, DON'T grit your teeth or try to use willpower to force it out of your mind. DON'T struggle with it.

Any fighting with the thought will only accentuate it and make it stronger, and you will end up becoming frustrated and upset. Don't risk losing the battle. Just simply drop the desire/thought from your field of attention.

Instead, give your full attention to your wellness vision and your bigger WHY. Remain immersed in these thoughts until you are completely calm.

It is simply a matter of learning HOW and WHERE to place your attention. Your wellness vision is a great point of focus for the challenging times when temptation is strong.

Old habits won't fall off overnight; give the process patience and commitment, and most importantly, stay inspired by your vision. Keep coming back to the WHY behind your actions.

HOW TO STOP EMOTIONAL EATING

Emotional eating and overeating are two of the worst things that you can do to your digestive system. Emotional eating happens when you want to be out of the moment or numb the feelings. It also happens when you forget the true purpose of your body. The bigger WHY for feeling good that we discussed in the chapter on wellness vision helps to identify the bigger idea behind your daily effort to support your body. Remembering the true purpose of your body helps you to treat it with love and care. Whenever you feel off track, think of your WHY and the things that you can't achieve without your body feeling healthy, at ease, and light. If you haven't already created your wellness vision and your WHY, please go back to Chapter 15 and do it now, before reading any further.

The issue of emotional eating almost always comes up when I work with women. Beautiful women who seem to have everything going for them complain about uncontrollable emotional eating and a draining sense of guilt afterward. When emotions take over — especially anxiety, worry, and stress — many of us turn to food for some grounding and reward. We know it is not right. We know that it is not the way to fix the situation. But, for some reason, it is damn hard to do what is right all of the time.

It is a well-known phenomenon that stress causes stronger cravings for sugary and fatty foods in many people. It is another survival mechanism that allowed our ancestors to make it through. To prepare for potential starvation periods, the human body was wired to stock up on energy reserves. High-sugar and high-fat foods were the best options.

However, times have changed and our stress comes less from chasing the prey (or potentially becoming one) and more from being mentally and emotionally overwhelmed. The body doesn't know the difference between emotionally- or physically-induced stress, so we respond to a stressful call or bad traffic the same way our ancestors would have responded to a tiger chasing them. Our adrenaline and cortisol levels shoot up, and we go into fight-or-flight mode and move away from rest and digest. Cravings hit shortly after.

The major difference, though, is that we don't have a shortage of food and don't have to run away from dangerous animals as our predecessors did. So cravings turned from a useful survival tool into a not-so-welcome side effect of stress.

I used to be drawn into the kitchen every time there was an e-mail I didn't want to write or a project I resented. Almonds and chocolate made things better for a few moments. The bad thing is that it would literally be just a few moments before I would feel guilty and unpleasantly full. It would always trigger digestive unease, bloating, and heaviness.

Recognizing this trend and making it a habit to breathe and say a short grace before eating (and snacking) made it a lot easier to recognize and prevent emotional eating. I still love almonds and chocolate, but now I eat them when I'm happy, not just when I am trying to avoid something.

Another thing that helped a lot was music. Music affects the way we feel and the way our nervous systems work.

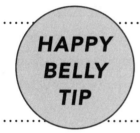

HAPPY BELLY TIP

Listening to your favorite tunes when you want to feel good is better for your digestion than reaching for a cookie.

Make a list of things that make you happy and relaxed and choose to create substitute behaviors. For example, instead of going out for a cupcake and a coffee to take a break from the computer, you can choose to take a walk while listening to your favorite song. You always have a choice to do what makes you happy short-term and is good for you long-term.

Come Back to the Breath

If you are having trouble with overeating and emotional eating, cultivate a regular meditation and yoga practice to put you in the moment.

Meditation and yoga can be superhelpful. Meditation and yoga are proven to lower cortisol levels and help create a better connection between our minds and our bodies. Slowly paced, mindfulness-based movement, such as yoga, helps you to increase awareness of emotions and to see how certain emotions can lead to cravings. Mindfulness gained in meditation acts as a "pause," as a safe padding between an arising emotion and your response. Having a "pause" allows you to make a choice and avoid reactive habitual behaviors. Choosing your actions versus being a slave to habits is a powerful transformation that creates freedom in your relationship with food.

First, you learn to do it on the mat, by being aware of your body and breath, and then it extends to all areas of your life. When you learn to stay mindful and present off the mat, in an uncomfortable, intense, or emotional situation in life, you can choose what is best for your body and keep yourself integrated with your wellness vision and goals.

Try meditating for a few minutes before each meal or when you feel that you are caught up in a whirlwind of emotions. The purpose is to ask your body if there is anything in particular you can provide that would support it at the current moment. You can download a short premeal meditation at www.spinachandyoga.com/resources.

Our body's needs change from day to day, especially in stressful situations. Our body tries its best to maintain a healthy balanced state in all situations. It uses feelings and sensations, including cravings, to communicate those needs to us, hoping we can meet them accordingly.

After a long, stressful day, a lot of us have a craving for something rich and sweet (chocolate or nuts, for example). This is how we interpret our body's need for *grounding* and *more energy*. A tired, stressed-out body needs to replenish energy and to cool down the nervous system. Cacao and sugar stimulate the entire system, creating an illusion of energy, while heavy nuts create grounding to calm down the nervous system.

While chocolate and nuts provide short-term relief, they are not ideal for a stressed-out, tired body and mind. The energy coming from stimulating substances such as chocolate, coffee (afternoon latte, anyone?), or even green tea is not real. It is borrowed. Real energy comes from sleep and relaxation. Stimulating substances put stress on the adrenal glands and excite the nervous system, preparing the body for a fight-or-flight situation. Nuts are healthy and have good fats that help us to feel more grounded, but they are quite heavy for a tired body to digest at the end of a long day.

A more sustainable way to help a stressed out and tired body is to take a few deep breaths, do a yoga nidra, and listen to calm music followed by an easy-to-digest dinner with a veggie soup or a seasonal stew. Over time, if you recognize your body's needs before cravings take over, causing you to mindlessly devour an entire box of cookies or a chocolate bar, you can save yourself a few pounds and an upset digestive system.

Mindful listening to the body through a mental body scan is one of the easiest ways to understand your body's needs. Relaxation, in its turn, helps to quiet a rambling mind so you can hear and understand your internal voice better. It is a skill that needs to be developed, as does any other skill. Practice makes perfect.

Sasha Loring,[39] an expert on emotional eating, offers a three-step approach to overcoming emotional eating and cravings that lead to excessive consumption. The first is examining the "wanting mind," the second is becoming more savvy about how your attention gets fixated on what you want, and the third is learning how to transform this fixation into an offering.

Examining the wanting mind means being aware of cravings. By observing desire itself and by letting it go again and again, you can bring a more settled and satisfying sense of equanimity into your life instead of being constantly subject to a never-ending series of desires. When the urge arises to eat for reasons that have nothing to do with hunger, remember to sit with yourself and tune in to what it is you really need in that moment. We are a society addicted to speed, and sometimes just sitting down and taking the time to "reset the inner compass" will provide the guidance you need.

IF YOU SLIP UP

Shame, guilt, disgust — what else do you feel toward yourself after giving in to temptation and stuffing your belly with not-so-good food? We tend to be pretty mean toward ourselves. If we spoke to our friends the way we talk to our bodies, we would not have any friends. No one in her right mind would put up with such a mean, angry, and demanding friend!

Negative emotions have a horrible effect on your body. They hinder digestion, create acidity, and adversely affect self-confidence and body image. They might have a worse effect than overeating or eating something bad. It is difficult to overcome negative feelings of failure and guilt after bingeing or slipping off the preferred menu. Harboring negative feelings toward yourself about bad choices can be worse than consuming the inferior food in the first place. The feeling of guilt is like double cursing the situation because the guilt is an emotional response that causes stress in the body, which leads to poor digestion or indigestion.

So what do you do with guilt and other negative feelings that can overwhelm you? Being kinder to your body doesn't mean being good to yourself and patting yourself on the back when you are being "good." It means being patient and kind to yourself when it is literally the last thing you want to do. Sometimes being kind is not easy when you feel horrible about your own actions such as overeating, drinking too much, or having forbidden foods.

After a binge, your natural urge might be to shower yourself with a rain of self-hatred, and then force yourself to starve or do a grueling workout. Take a look at this set of actions from the point of view of your body: you forcefully stuffed it past the comfort zone, called it bad names, bullied it, and then tortured it with exhausting exercise.

If your partner or a friend were to treat you that way, how would you feel about her? You probably wouldn't trust her very much in the future, would you? So our body too stops trusting that we are on the same team.

Instead, a kinder action after a binge would be to reduce the negative effects of the action, figure out its cause, and most importantly, ask for forgiveness from your body. While you can't fully undo what has been done, you can do a few things to help your body deal with the binge with fewer negative consequences. Take a walk outside, drink some ginger tea, skip the next meal if your stomach still feels heavy or have a light nourishing meal such as chicken rice soup or veggie soup, get an acupuncture or reflexology treatment, do a deep relaxation, or meditate on forgiveness.

Remember: progress, not perfection!

You and I can choose how to feel at any moment.

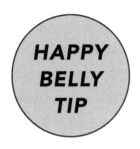

When you feel bad after slipping up and failing, come back to your vision for inspiration; don't stay stuck on guilt and shame. Get clear on how you want to feel in your body and focus on creating those feelings with every breath.

There is always a reality where you feel happy, content, calm. It is just a matter of stepping into it. You don't have to do anything to deserve feeling good; you just need to actively choose the state of being that you want to experience. The more you focus on how you want to feel and look, the easier and more inspired you will feel to create actions that support that vision.

....

chapter 22

YOU ARE UNIQUE

Bef_ore rushing to change your diet, let's get clear on something. Your body is unique. You are different from me and from everyone else on planet Earth. Your body, your mind, your emotions, your views, your life, your perceptions of stress, and your habits make up a unique microcosm that is YOU. As a result, your digestive system is unique too. It needs a unique approach to heal. You are the only one who can find that ideal approach. Things that work for some other people might not work for you, and that is fine. It doesn't mean that something is wrong with you. It just means that you are unique.

There are many different approaches to food and nutrition: vegan, raw, paleo, macrobiotic, gluten- and dairy-free, ayurvedic, and so on. Each approach has a good number of followers who swear by it. Usually, ardent followers attribute their weight loss success, health breakthroughs and other positive results to their diet of choice. While we hear about the wonderful success stories, all the failures stay behind the scenes. We rarely hear stories about people whose skin and digestive issues didn't clear up after going gluten-free or who didn't lose weight after adopting a vegan diet. No one wants to share failures. As a result, every diet seems to work for many people. Every diet has lots of back-up success stories, and very few recorded failures. All diets sound as if they would work for you if only you could decide which one to follow.

I am not writing this to announce the new best diet. I am not a doctor and won't tell you which diet is best for your body. Your doctor probably won't either. I am writing this to remind you that you are the only person who can decide which approach to nutrition is right for you.

Often, the biggest breakthroughs occur when we let go of the desire to find a quick fix, a magic pill, or a miraculous herb and turn internally for guidance. I grew to accept the idea of uncertainty and be okay with not knowing everything. Our environment, food policies, and scientific findings are always shifting and changing. The skill that serves best is to stay flexible and attentive to the shifts. Instead of being strict, and judgmental, try to flow, be curious, treat everything as an experiment, and enjoy the process of change.

A lot of information on what to eat or not to eat is based on personal experience. Most health food claims are not supported by any research. And, unfortunately, many holistic doctors don't agree with each other when it comes to deciding on the best diet or supplements.

I think it happens because we tend to think that we are all the same. The assumption is that your body is the same as everyone else's body. If my body feels great on any particular diet, then you will feel great on it too. This leads to recommendations based on personal experience, which might apply to your body or it might not, just as size 7 shoes fit me, but might not fit you.

Your Body Is Your Guide—Listen

You live inside your body—not me, not some other expert, nutritionist, or doctor. While it is helpful and oftentimes very interesting to review research, learn about new approaches, and listen to other people's experiences, your body is unique and what works for others might not work for you. So, get all the info you can, but rely on the cues from your body to make a final decision. Being too much in your head makes it hard to be in your body. From time to time, it's good to let go of all the articles and books that you read and check in with your body. Touch it, breathe, talk with it, and listen. Create a collaboration of outer and inner wisdom.

WHEN YOU FEEL OVERWHELMED AND CONFLICTED

There are lots of health- and fitness-related articles out there. If our grandparents and parents had to put in effort to find health-related resources, we have to put in the effort to protect ourselves from health-related information overload.

You would think that having so much information at hand would turn us into the healthiest nation ever, but quite the opposite: we are fatter than ever and suffering from chronic disease and auto-immune malfunction.

Too much information on health and wellness can lead to anxiety and lack of motivation to follow any of the often-conflicting advice. How are you supposed to choose which advice to follow if you want to increase your energy? Someone is telling you to go raw, another expert is banning sugar and coffee, someone else offers energy-boosting exercise. But you also read that some exercise depletes energy and that our body needs sugars and that raw foods are harder to digest. It can get pretty confusing, to say the least.

Just as eating in a rush without chewing leads to indigestion and a bloated belly, skimming through a ton of articles without taking time to process and absorb information will lead to misunderstanding and a bloated head.

The Hardest Thing You Have to Do to Feel Great in Your Body: Listen and Trust Your Body's Wisdom

The truth is there is no universal rule for what to eat and how much to exercise that perfectly fits every woman out there. I am not even talking about every person out there. Stop searching for it! Save your time and effort!

One of the most important skills that we are not being taught is listening and understanding our body. We are taught to do the research, to trust specialists, to put the responsibility for our well-being into the hands of professionals. We are not encouraged, after childhood, to check in with our body, to have an internal dialogue, to build a trusting relationship between our body and mind.

Instead, our mind is supposed to control our body through willpower and if it fails to do so, it is our weakness, our failure.

Unfortunately, living in a mind-controlled, willpower-based relationship with ourselves is tiring, and most of all it often creates a deep internal conflict. Over time, this conflict leads to binges, self-loathing, cheat days (who exactly are we cheating?), and the feeling that every meal should be calculated in terms of calories, carbs, fats, and protein ratios, and bloating versus nonbloating foods. This approach forbids playfulness, freedom, relaxation, and spontaneity.

If you like being a mathematician in your kitchen, good for you! I much prefer going with the flow and not feeling squeezed into the tight frames of dos and don'ts.

I bet you would rather not stress out about going to a restaurant with friends because you are afraid that there won't be anything on the menu that you can eat. You would rather not be afraid of food and not keep in mind the exact amount of carbs, proteins, and fats of all the foods you ate throughout the day. Plus, I want to share a little—but superimportant—secret here. *Whenever you are in a stressed-out, overwhelmed, or uncertain state about your food, no matter what's on your plate, it won't be digested well.*

So what's the solution? How does all of this translate into what you should eat and how often you should exercise? Learn to ask and trust your body. Ask your body, when did it feel its best? What was around? What did you eat?

It all goes back to living in alignment with your ideal vision of yourself. If you know how you want to feel and look, and why, it is not hard to know what will get you there. Only you can choose a diet that is nourishing and healing and not controlling and restricting.

The hardest part is doing what your body tells you is the right thing and letting go of constantly comparing your diet and exercise regimen to others in the hope of finding something more effective.

Here is where the importance of having a clear wellness vision comes in. You need to have that bright picture of how you want to feel and look and a clear understanding of WHY you want your wellness vision to be a reality.

Whenever you feel off track or start questioning your diet or exercise routine, do this little trick: come back to your wellness vision. See how you look and feel there. See yourself moving through your regular activities looking and feeling this way: walking the streets, writing, working, interacting with people. Connect with that ideal picture of yourself. And then ask your ideal self what she does to feel that way, what she eats, what gets her inspired, what she enjoys doing for exercise. It will help to realign your daily actions with your ideal image. If you have trouble imagining that, download a guided wellness vision meditation from www.spinachandyoga.com/resources.

A CURE FOR AN OVERWHELMED, HEALTH-SEEKING WARRIOR

Here are a few guidelines that might help you to navigate the overabundance of health and wellness information and to start your own health transformation without overstressing.

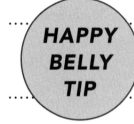

HAPPY BELLY TIP

Remember: you already know more than you realize! Trust your inner expert!

- **Before Googling, ask yourself the question to which you seek an answer.** There's a good chance you already know it. For example, if you are wondering how to reduce bloating or increase energy, what has worked for you in the past? Close your eyes and ask your body the question. Listen to what your body has to say. An answer to increasing energy might be very simple, such as, "Dude, put me to sleep!" or "Let's go for a walk," or "I would really appreciate some stretches now." Ask yourself first! If there is no good answer, then try Google.

- **Limit research to two to three articles and give yourself time to digest and assimilate information.** You know that you can't rush digestion in your belly without creating indigestion, so why would you want to rush digestion in your brain? You skim through the articles without pausing to think and to see how this information applies to your life. Let it sink in, simmer, become a part of you, and then, when it is fully assimilated, you can use it to build up to your desired outcomes. Also, pay attention to the research supporting the claims in the article. Who paid for the research? What is the background of the author? Is there any hidden underlying agenda?

- **Choose just one thing to change at a time.** Experiments are effective when you keep variables to a minimum and observe the true "cause and effect" in action. Don't try to revamp your entire lifestyle in one week. Slow down and enjoy the ride. Listen to your body's feedback and allow time and space for constant evolution.

- **Talk it through with a friend or with a coach.** Write or talk about the benefits and disadvantages of changing your habits. Find out what worked for your friends and why. Get a perspective from a human being—not just the Internet. Brainstorm and play with new ideas.

Avoid information pollution and be picky about what you let in. Most importantly, never try to search for the *final truth*. It is not there. Or to be more exact, it will be different for every person, for every day, for every climate, for every season, and every level of physical and emotional stress. There are millions of variations for the *final truth*. Be easy on yourself and instead of trying to be absolute in your commitments to any particular food and perfect in your way of following any particular diet, try to be aware of your body's cues and brave enough to let go of the beliefs that are not serving you anymore.

Keep in mind that we are all in search of an *optimal* nutrition plan that allows us to be at a healthy weight easily and gives us lots of energy. Ideally, it would also leave us feeling nourished both physically and emotionally.

It is not an invitation to eat everything that you see in the supermarket. It is an invitation to be mindful and to stay flexible.

Make a decision about how you want to feel on a daily basis and pay attention to the food that your body gravitates to. Be honest when paying attention.

 **HAPPY BELLY TIP** Differentiate between old patterns, habits, and emotions and what your body is telling you.

Being paranoid about food is going to hurt you more than the food. Being fearful is not conducive to healing your digestion or any other part of your body

chapter 24

AYURVEDA—ANCIENT WISDOM FOR MODERN HEALTH

A yurveda, an ancient Indian science of life and health, helped me appreciate my unique needs and understand my digestive system better. It gave me tools to heal my belly and to eliminate the most aggravating foods and habits. While I don't consider myself an ayurvedic expert, I will share some main ayurvedic principles that have made a huge difference for me and my clients.

It is believed that ayurveda originated in India over 5,000 years ago. Establishing and maintaining balance in the body, mind, and emotions is the main focus of ayurvedic medicine. Diet, lifestyle, exercise, cleansing, and herbal remedies are the main tools of ayurveda.

HOW IS AYURVEDA DIFFERENT FROM MODERN MEDICINE?

In ayurveda, every individual is unique, and there is no diet or lifestyle routine that works for everyone.

Digestion in ayurveda is considered a cornerstone of good vibrant health. A lot of attention is given to strengthening digestion and educating people to maintain a balanced digestive fire (*agni*) that creates good health, energy, and a feeling of lightness.

Prevention is key. Ayurveda focuses on providing specific advice and guidance on how to maintain physical and emotional health.

Food and lifestyle routines are considered the most important medicine. If you go to an ayurvedic doctor with a complaint, you are more likely to leave with a recipe than with a prescription for pills.

HOW DOES AYURVEDA WORK?

Ayurveda is based on the principle of three *doshas* or mind-body constitutions. Doshas are the energies that make up every individual and that perform different physiological functions in the body.

This is a very simplistic introduction of ayurveda and dosha types. If it strikes a chord with you, you can learn more in the wonderful books of Dr. Vasant Lad, Dr. Claudia Welch, Dr. Robert Svoboda, and Dr. David Frawley, among many others.

The three dosha types are:

1. **Vata Dosha.** Vata controls bodily functions associated with motion, including blood circulation, breathing, blinking, and the heartbeat. When in balance, there is creativity and vitality. When out of balance, there can be fear and anxiety.

2. **Pitta Dosha.** Pitta controls the body's metabolic systems, including digestion, absorption, nutrition, and the body's temperature. When in balance, pitta leads to contentment and

intelligence. When it is out of balance, it can cause irritation and anger.

3. Kapha Dosha. Kapha controls growth in the body. It supplies water to all body parts, moisturizes the skin, and maintains the immune system. When kapha is in balance, it is expressed as love and forgiveness. When it is out of balance, it can lead to insecurity, weight gain, and envy.

Everybody has all three doshas, but usually one or two dominate. The level of dominance of the various doshas determines one's physiological and personality traits, as well as general likes and dislikes.

The ayurvedic approach uses your body type and your digestive tendencies to create a personalized diet. Not knowing your body type and not understanding the nature of your needs leads to health problems including digestive disorders. The wrong way of approaching your body type can throw you out of balance and keep you in a state of continual disequilibrium, which plants the seeds for disease. Generalizing and giving everyone the same advice does not work, according to ayurveda.

Each mind/body type is considered to exhibit the characteristics listed below.

- **Characteristics of vata-predominant types:** creative; quick to learn and grasp new knowledge but also quick to forget; slender, tall; fast walker; tendency to cold hands and feet; discomfort in cold climates; excitable, lively, fun personality; changeable moods; irregular daily routine; high energy in short bursts; tendency to tire easily and to overexert; full of joy and enthusiasm when in balance; responds to stress with fear, worry, and anxiety, especially when out of balance; tendency to act on impulse; and often have racing, disjointed thoughts. Vata-predominant types often have dry skin and dry hair and don't perspire much.

- **Characteristics of pitta-predominant types:** medium physique, strong, well-built; sharp mind, good concentration powers; orderly, focused; assertive, self-confident, and entrepreneurial at their best; aggressive, demanding, pushy when out of balance; competitive, enjoy challenges; passionate and romantic; strong digestion, strong appetite, get irritated if they have to miss or wait for a meal; when under stress, pittas become irritated and angry; skin fair or reddish, often with freckles, sunburns easily; uncomfortable in sun or hot weather, heat makes them very tired; perspire a lot; good public speakers; they generally demonstrate good management and leadership ability but they also can become authoritarian, and may be subject to temper tantrums, impatience, and anger; typical physical problems include rashes or inflammations of the skin, acne, boils, skin cancer, ulcers, heartburn, acid stomach, insomnia, dry or burning eyes.

- **Characteristics of kapha-predominant types:** easygoing, relaxed, slow-paced; affectionate and loving; forgiving, compassionate, nonjudgmental nature; stable and reliable; faithful; physically strong and with a sturdy, heavier build; have the most energy of all constitutions, but Kaphas are steady and enduring; slow of speech, slower to learn, but have an outstanding long-term memory; soft hair and skin; tendency to have large "soft" eyes and a low, soft voice; tend toward being overweight; may also suffer from sluggish digestion; prone to depression; more self-sufficient; gentle, and essentially have an undemanding approach to life; excellent health, and a good immune system. They are very calm and strive to maintain harmony and peace in their surroundings. They are not easily upset and can provide stability for others. But kapha-pedominant types tend to be possessive and hold on to things; they don't like cold, damp weather; and their physical problems include colds and congestion. They often suffer from sinus headaches; respiratory problems including asthma, allergies, and atherosclerosis (hardening of the arteries).

How Do I Determine My Type?

Most books and websites on ayurveda will offer questionnaires that can be used to determine your mind/body constitution. My favorite one is offered by Holistic Online, at http://www. holisticonline.com/ayurveda/w_ayurveda-dtest1.htm, which is detailed and thorough. Most questionnaires are very similar and will provide somewhat similar results. Please keep in mind that shorter questionnaires will give more generalized and approximate results. Also, your body changes with age, seasons, and life situations, so the results will change as well. Using a few different questionnaires will give you a more definitive result for your dosha type. If you are serious about ayurveda, it is best to see a qualified ayurvedic practitioner.

Once you know and understand your body type, try to follow the diet and lifestyle routine that fits your mind/body constitution.

Here are some general guidelines for each type.

- **General health tips for vata types.** Maintain regular habits and try to eat and sleep at the same time every night. Get enough rest and choose foods that are warm, cooked, nourishing, and easy to digest. Sweet berries, sweet juicy fruits, small beans, grains such as rice and quinoa, and all nuts (soaked) and organic and fresh dairy products (if you do not have a sensitivity to dairy) are generally good choices for vata types. Exercise intensity should be moderate. A more meditative yoga, tai chi, walking, and swimming are all good. Avoid strenuous and frantic activities.

- **General health tips for pitta types.** It's important for pittas to keep cool by avoiding overexposure to direct sunlight and fried and spicy foods. Avoid alcohol and tobacco, overworking, and overheating. When aggravated, pitta types are susceptible to feeling negative emotions such as hostility, hatred, intolerance, and jealousy. Choose fresh vegetables and fruits that are watery and sweet, especially cherries, mangoes, cucumbers, watermelon, and avocado. Enjoy salads with dark greens such as arugula, dandelions, and kale. Avoid conflicts. Cultivate self-acceptance, surrender, letting go, and kindness to self and others.

- **General health tips for kapha types.** It's important to be active on a daily basis as kapha types are prone to sluggishness, depression, and excess weight. Getting out of the house and actively seeking new experiences is also recommended. Be receptive to change and try to be intentional in implementing life-enhancing actions. Choose foods that are light, warm, and spicy. Tea with dried ginger and lemon is a great pick-me-up for kaphas. Avoid heavy, oily foods, and processed sugars, which are harmful to kaphas. Use lots of spices such as black pepper, ginger, cumin, chili, and lots of bitter dark greens.

Ayurveda and Your Belly

According to ayurveda, digestion is the cornerstone of health. A huge part of this ancient tradition is focused on what to eat, how to cook it, what is best for different body types, and what to do when your digestion is off.

You don't need to become proficient in ayurveda, dosha types, or read ancient texts to benefit from core ayurvedic principles. These principles are simple but very powerful. Some of them might completely change the way you look at food, while others will be helpful in understanding why your digestion is acting up now.

chapter 25

AYURVEDIC PRINCIPLES AND HOW TO USE THEM TO IMPROVE DIGESTION

Ayurveda is a very elaborate science that covers diet, lifestyle, herbs, thought processes, relationships, and even surgery. We will look only at the small aspect of it that is related to digestion.

These are the principles we will cover:

1. Balance is the ultimate goal: like increases like and opposites create balance.

2. All food can be broken down into harder or easier to digest.

3. Food is information. Every food and herb has its own personality that affects you when you eat it.

4. You are unique; your diet should be unique to you.

5. Teas and herbs can be very healing and may be used to improve digestion and soothe the gut.

6. Appropriate movement for your type can be used to improve digestion, metabolism, and make elimination more efficient.

Keep in mind that a diet and lifestyle that worked thousands of years ago in another country are not guaranteed to work in today's Western world. We have to account for our environment, lifestyle, responsibilities, and desires. We can use past knowledge for guidance, inspiration, principles, and lessons. But in the end, it is okay to change things, to adapt them to *you*, and not feel bad about letting go of the way things were done thousands of years ago.

While my way of explaining ayurveda may be very simplified and non-traditional, it is the first step in learning this amazing science. Often simplicity is the key to not overloading our already-overstimulated brain. These principles have worked for many of my clients; I hope they will work for you as well.

LIKE INCREASES LIKE AND OPPOSITES CREATE BALANCE

A body in a balanced state is healthy and happy. Any kind of a disease, an unpleasant symptom, or a negative state of being is a sign of imbalance. The purpose of food, activities, exercise, and herbs is to re-create and maintain balance.

We are constantly interacting with our environment and everything we touch, eat, or do has an effect on us. We are never separate in our own little world, even if it might seem so sometimes. We are in a constant state of change and flowing from one state to another. The ability to balance and the knowledge of what needs to be balanced grows from a deep awareness of your internal state.

A practitioner of ayurveda, a person who practices the principles of ayurveda in daily living, is more likely to be using the magic of balancing, not the curse of living with restrictions. Balancing a heavy meal with spices that improve digestion, balancing a feeling of sluggishness with tastes that get the blood moving and ideas flowing, using intelligent nourishing foods and herbs to balance out depletion from stress—all is done to stay in equilibrium. Your balanced spot is unique and determined by your inborn constitution and the living environment with which you interact. Staying balanced, for someone who suffers from bloating and constipation, will require a different set of daily practices and foods than what is needed by someone suffering from diarrhea.

Through daily internal dialogue with your body you become more aware of how your body feels and what it needs. You also become more in tune with the qualities and effects of certain foods, herbs, and actions. Ayurvedic books can be great guides at the beginning of the journey. What can be better than using the wisdom of those who have gone through the journey before and were kind enough to share information?

However, most likely you won't be learning the qualities and effects of every single food at the food store, the herbs you use, and the spices you like. At a certain point, you will be taking the initiative of consulting your own senses and awareness, since reaching for a book every time you put something in your body is a bit restricting. It will become more intuitive and automatic over time.

Knowledge of ayurveda helps to turn your kitchen into a magical lab where you create balance with a touch of spice, a sprinkle of lime juice, and a timely tea.

Example of Using Opposites to Create Balance

On rainy, foggy, gloomy days, it is common to feel sleepy, sluggish, puffy, and slow. Changes in the weather always lead to changes in our bodies. Our microcosm always interacts with macrocosm outside us. To balance the heaviness and wetness of the weather, we can use food, movement, and spices to create balance. Getting lots of movement and eating warm, light, and spicy foods can be a great counterbalancing prescription. Eating beans and roasted veggies while avoiding heavy, cold, and creamy stuff is good for rainy days. Hot water with lemon and some cinnamon can help reenergize. In general, warming spices are great on cooler days. Use ginger, turmeric, cinnamon, and cloves! Wearing bright colors, such as red, yellow, and orange, to counteract gray and dull weather is another great way to bring yourself in balance.

Another example of using opposite qualities to create balance is eating a heavy, oily, and cold avocado with warming black pepper or chilies, sprinkled with lime juice to increase digestive juices, and salt, which is hot by nature. This will prevent the avocado's coldness and heaviness from creating mucus, a "runny nose," and a clogging effect.

A cold, potentially mucus-forming ice cream can still be enjoyed during a hot day without too many negative effects if sprinkled with warming cinnamon and cardamom and followed with fresh ginger tea. The heating effects of chocolate can be diminished by using cooling herbs such as cardamon, rose hip, or fennel tea.

One of the easiest ways to balance the qualities and effects of your meals is to understand the six tastes.

BALANCE OF TASTES

In ayurveda, food is classified by six tastes: sweet, sour, salty, bitter, pungent, and astringent.

Each taste has a specific effect on the body. If you have too much or too little of a certain taste, the body becomes imbalanced. When tastes are in balance, we have fewer cravings, better digestion, and a greater sense of satisfaction.

Usually our body lets us know that one of the tastes is missing or that there is an internal imbalance with cravings.

HAPPY BELLY TIP

Our body experiences cravings when something is missing, whether it is a physical microelement, a kind emotion, or a fulfilling role in society.

For example, according to ayurveda, *love* and *compassion* are sweet, so if you are missing one of them in your day-to-day life, you might experience cravings for sweets to make up for the missing piece. Your body has to get sweetness, in whatever form it comes, one way or the other to stay balanced. One of the strategies to stay in balance and avoid cravings is to include all six ayurvedic tastes into every meal.

Certain tastes help stimulate digestion and overabundance of others can create heaviness, stagnation, and toxins. In general, our Western diet is very predominant in sweet, salty, and sour tastes but severely lacks liver-cleansing bitter. Once you understand the six tastes, it will be easier to balance your meals and hopefully, your digestion.

According to ayurveda, a healthy balance of the six tastes creates harmony in the body, while the predominance of one of the tastes can throw the entire system off balance. Ever feel sleepy and heavy after a hearty portion of tiramisu? This is the effect that too much "sweet taste" can have on the system if it is not balanced. Each taste feeds our mind, body, and senses in a unique way.

Here is an overview of the six tastes and their effects,

summarized from *Eat Taste Heal: An Ayurvedic Cookbook for Modern Living* by Thomas Yarema and Daniel Rhoda.[40]

Sweet

- Qualities: Sweet taste is heavy, oily, moist, and cooling by nature.

- Effects: Sweet foods enhance strength, longevity, and stability. Sweet tastes naturally increase moisture and weight in the body, if you overindulge. Sweet also relieves burning sensations and thirst, and has beneficial effects on the skin and hair. It is a good choice if you are feeling ungrounded and agitated. When you feel nervous or ungrounded you intuitively reach for a sweet taste to ground. It doesn't have to be cookies; you can satisfy that craving for grounding with roasted beets, squash, or a grain dish. If you are always craving sweets and your blood sugar levels are unbalanced, you can create balance with a "sweet" taste of proteins which will stabilize blood sugar.

- Sources: All sweet fruits, grains, dairy, nuts, and most proteins such as chicken and fish. It is not necessarily sugary but it is always good-tasting and nourishing.

Sour

- Qualities: Sour taste is hot, light, and moist by nature.

- Effects: Sour stimulates digestion, helps circulation and elimination, nourishes and energizes the body, strengthens the heart, relieves thirst, maintains acidity, sharpens the senses, and helps extract minerals such as iron from food. In excess, it may result in heartburn. Since sours help digestion, it is a good idea to include a slice of lime or some lactofermented vegetables at every meal.

- Sources: It is commonly found in citrus fruits such as lemon and limes; sour dairy products such as yogurt, cheese, and sour cream; and fermented substances including wine, vinegar, pickles, sauerkraut, and lactofermented vegetables.

Salty

- Qualities: Salty taste is heavy and moist (oily) by nature.

- Effects: Salty taste improves the flavor of food, stimulates digestion, lubricates tissues, maintains mineral balance, aids in the elimination of wastes, and calms the nerves. Salty taste has a drying quality in the mouth, but it is moistening internally and has a water-retaining quality. Due to its tendency to attract water, it helps balance out electrolytes and improves the radiance of the skin. When you are dehydrated or going on a hike in the sun, make a homemade electrolyte drink with a pinch of salt, lime juice, and honey.

- Sources: Good sources include sea salt and rock salt; sea vegetables such as seaweed and kelp; and foods to which large amounts of salt are added such as nuts, chips, and pickles.

Pungent

- Qualities: Pungent taste is the hottest of all tastes and also possesses dry and light qualities.

- Effects: Pungent taste stimulates digestion, clears the sinuses, promotes sweating and detoxification, aids circulation, improves metabolism, and relieves muscle pain. It also increases clarity and perception. When you feel sleepy or sluggish, add some pungent taste to your food. Cayenne or chili will quickly wake you up!

- Sources: It is found in certain vegetables such as chili peppers, radishes, garlic, and onions, and in spices such as black pepper, ginger, cayenne, and mustard.

Bitter

- Qualities: Bitter is light, cooling, and dry by nature.
- Effects: The bitter taste is lacking in the Western diet. While bitter taste is rarely eaten alone, it stimulates the appetite and helps bring out the flavor of the other tastes. Bitter taste is a powerful detoxifying agent, and has antibiotic, antiparasitic, and antiseptic qualities. It is also helpful in reducing weight, water retention, skin rashes, fever, burning sensations, and nausea. Make sure to get dark leafy greens at least once a day!

- Sources: It is found in green leafy vegetables such as spinach, kale, and green cabbage and in other vegetables, including zucchini and eggplant; other sources include herbs and spices such as turmeric, fenugreek, and dandelion root; coffee and tea; and certain fruits such as grapefruit, olives, and bitter melon.

Astringent

- Qualities: Astringent is dry, cooling, and heavy by nature.

- It is the least common of all six. Astringent taste is classified more in relation to its effect on the tongue than its actual taste. It creates a puckering sensation in the mouth (such as with cranberries) or a dry, chalky feeling (such as with many varieties of bean). Foods such as broccoli or cauliflower have a mildly astringent taste that is less detectable.

- Effects: Astringent is thought to soothe ulcers and improve clotting. Too much makes a person physically and emotionally inflexible. It can cause constipation. Eating astringent foods on an empty stomach can increase bloating in people with a sensitive digestion.

- Sources: It can be found in legumes such as chickpeas and lentils; fruits, including cranberries, pomegranates, green bananas and dried fruit; vegetables such as alfalfa sprouts, broccoli, cauliflower, artichoke, asparagus, green beans, and turnips; grains such as rye, buckwheat, and quinoa; spices and herbs, including turmeric and marjoram; coffee, and tea.

Ayurvedic nutrition recommends including all six in each meal, while favoring those tastes that balance out your particular constitution and seasonal changes. Keep the concept of tastes and their effects on your body in the back of your mind to address any negative emotions or physical complaints such as being tired or irritated.

PRESERVING ENERGY

Digestion is an energy-consuming task for the body. Easy-to-digest foods will leave more energy in the body to do other things. Hard-to-digest foods might leave you very little energy to do other things. This idea is simple, but it is key to feeling light and clear. When tired or short on time, eat easy-to-digest food that takes little effort to digest and assimilate.

Certain foods require less energy to be digested. Monomeals are among easy-to-digest nourishing meals. Ancient cultures and countries still following old cultural traditions have a lesson to teach us about monomeals.

There is a big difference between nutritionally rich foods and the ones that are easy to digest and will make your stomach feel good. Ideally, one's diet should consist of nutritionally rich food that is easy to digest. It will mean different things for different people, depending on their digestion strength.

When your digestion is weak, you might not be able to digest some nutritionally rich foods. For example, a health bar might be made out of the best ingredients and have lots of vegan protein, fiber, omegas, and other goodies, but you may feel bloated and gassy after eating it. A similar situation will be true for some people with IBS who will react to fiber-rich raw vegetables or high-fat coconut even though they are nutritionally great.

In the ayurvedic tradition there is a saying that a person with a strong digestion can get benefits and nutrition from poison, while someone with a very weak digestion might feel sick even after drinking a pure health nectar. The health of our digestion determines how we break down food and absorb the nutrients or whether we absorb any at all.

If your digestion is weak, ayurveda has a few great tips and recipes that can help strengthen it. The key principle of strengthening digestion is letting it rest from hard-to-digest foods and helping the cleansing or restoration process with herbs. Soups are one of the easier-to-digest foods.

In most countries soup is a staple food—a food that is served on most days of the week and provides a large chunk of nutrition. In India, sambar, kitchari, and different varieties of dhals rule the kitchen. In Russia everyone loves borscht. Thai and Vietnamese kitchens boast yummy coconut stews and soups. The Japanese seem to live on miso soup and its varieties. And Koreans enjoy congee regularly. What is it about a warm, liquid-based meal that ancient cultures knew and that sandwich-eating Americans are missing? There are a few things that make soup an ideal monomeal that can boost your diet with vitamins and minerals while reducing indigestion aftereffects.

- Soups provide easily available nutrition and are easier to digest than most other forms of food. Liquid food limits strain on your digestive system. Your body absorbs liquids easily, and they don't irritate the digestive tract.

- Soups promote healthy elimination. Warm food increases blood circulation to your abdominal organs and helps to stimulate elimination. Most vegetarian soups, especially if small-bean-based or lentil-based, will provide a lot of fiber that many of us are lacking.

- Soups are easy and quick to make. What's easier than just throwing everything in one pot and letting it simmer?

Soaking beans, grains, and lentils overnight will speed up the process even more!

- Soups will let your digestive system recuperate. Liquid-based meals let digestive systems rest, help to eliminate toxins, and help to clear heavy, food-induced, mental fog. The reduction of stress or strain on the digestive system can often alleviate nausea, constipation, and diarrhea in people dealing with digestive conditions.

I bet if you have paid attention to your body after having a warm vegetarian soup, you noticed that your body gets a boost of energy, your tummy feels warm and happy, and, if you eat it often enough, there are no issues with irregular elimination.

Soup is one of my favorite things to cook and to eat. It's easy to make a power food with soups by using all kinds of seasonal vegetables and spices. It will never get boring if you use your creativity and try new ingredients. Soups also last for a few days in the fridge and will provide a wholesome meal when you are short on time. While eating leftover food is not ideal, let's be realistic — our life often makes cooking three meals a day impossible.

If you need to reduce your anxiety level, and along the way would like to improve your digestion, having a vegetarian, or even a simple soup with chicken or fish several times a week is an easy way to do it. Mung bean or thin lentil soups are among the best choices. Wild fish and vegetable or chicken and vegetable soups are also great.

In the ayurvedic tradition, kitchari is considered one of the most healing, balancing, nourishing, and digestion-friendly dishes. I think it is a great dish to experiment with when you are trying to find foods that do well in your stomach. For kitchari and other delicious soup recipes, go to www.spinachandyoga.com/recipes and check out the Kitchari recipe in the color insert.

Our body has an incredible healing capacity. We just need to create a favorable environment for the healing to take place. Whether you make a classic kitchari or a favorite hearty lentil soup, you will get a necessary dose of protein and fiber, along with iron, while keeping fat levels in check.

Note of Caution

Most people feel better within a couple of days on an easy-to-digest diet. So what do they do? They go and celebrate with a cookie or some chocolate with nuts—or worse, with a burger and fries. When you feel better, it's a sign that you are moving in the direction of healing, but it doesn't mean that your intestines are healed. It takes time — usually two to six weeks, depending on the severity of the issue.

Imagine a cut on your foot. Once your body forms an initial cover for the wound, you don't consider it fully healed yet, even though the pain may have diminished. The same process works on the inside. You need to give your body time to heal the inflammation and let the irritation and internal sore fully recover.

Time is your friend on this one! So stick with easy-to-digest foods until you feel 100 percent, at least for 2–3 weeks. After that, keep up with easy-to-digest foods for most dinners during the week.

EASIER-TO-DIGEST SUBSTITUTES

If you are trying to heal your gut, it doesn't mean that you should rely only on kitchari and soups. As long as you simplify the recipes and keep the ingredients anti-inflammatory and healthy, your belly should be happy.

According to nutritionist Dana James, food allergies and sensitivities are on the rise. Gluten, processed sugar, and dairy are on top of the list of irritating, gut-wrenching foods. More people are also becoming wary of consuming factory-produced animal products, whether due to the animal rights movement or due to the unhealthy diet that farm animals are being fed. As a result, I get a lot of questions on what to use as substitutes for old-time kitchen staples such as butter, sugar, flour, cream, milk, eggs, and margarine.

Fortunately, with a huge variety of foods from all over the world available online and at most health food stores, with a bit of research and creativity, you can replace all of the above without giving up on a taste, even while most often adding nutrients. Keeping to a healing, nourishing diet is not that difficult. You can download a list of healthy substitutes at www.spinachandyoga.com/resources.

If you decide to do a food sensitivity test to see what foods your digestive system is having a hard time with and the test comes back with multiple foods, don't try to eliminate all those foods. Focus on eliminating the foods that you are strongly sensitive to—such as dairy, gluten, and soy—and embarking on a self-healing regimen of herbs, happy thoughts, stress-reduction, and mindful, clean eating.

For example, I tested sensitive to a lot of foods including broccoli, eggplant, cabbage, almonds, peppers, onion, and garlic. Excluding the entire list would have left me with very few things to eat. Instead of overwhelming myself and stressing out by excluding everything, I opted for excluding the main trigger foods and paying close attention to how I felt after occasionally having cabbage, for example. Just as expected, my body didn't show a negative response to the veggies as long as I chewed them well, didn't have too much raw broccoli or cabbage, and had them primarily during the midday meals when digestion is the strongest.

The beauty of living in the age of the Internet is that there are lots of websites and blogs created by people who have food sensitivities. They've done your legwork for you by collecting recipes free of gluten, dairy, eggs, and nuts. All you have to do is search, bookmark, and start cooking with new foods so you don't feel deprived. You can bake delicious cookies without relying on sugar, butter, and chocolate. Make creamy soups without dairy, and create a party-pleasing dinner without triggering your body into an array of fatigue and GI problems for the next week.

For a Happy Belly list of my favorite must-have kitchen substitutes for baking, sauces, and dressings, please go to www. spinachandyoga.com/resources.

Some foods that are considered healthy may be too hard for a weak and sensitive gut.

"HEALTHY" SNACKS THAT MAY UPSET YOUR TUMMY

Nuts. One of the favorite snacks in North America, but unfortunately, nuts can be drying for the digestive system, hard to digest, and too heavy for most people. Americans eat more nuts than most other nations. Peanuts, almonds, pistachios, macadamia, Brazil nuts—the varieties and quantities are endless. Nuts are too expensive in most other countries to have them on a daily basis, but in the United States and Canada, they have become a go-to snack. While nuts are amazing in terms of nutrients, nutrients on their own are not what should determine whether you eat something. It is whether you can digest the product and absorb all those nutrients. If you can't digest it, no matter what it is, you shouldn't overload on it. Roasted nuts, found at most stores, are dry, heavy, oily, and hard to digest, according to ayurveda. They can aggravate a weak digestive system. To make nuts more digestible, ayurveda advises consumers to purchase fresh nuts (almonds are the best choice), and soak them for 8 to 36 hours. Soaking nuts rehydrates them, reduces phytic acid, which can irritate the stomach, and increases life energy (prana). Phytic acid binds to minerals such as zinc, iron, magnesium, calcium, chromium, and manganese in the gastrointestinal tract, unless it's reduced or nullified by soaking, sprouting, and/or fermentation. Bound minerals generally cannot be absorbed in the intestine, and too many bound minerals can lead to mineral deficiencies. Once the nuts have soaked, peel off the skin and enjoy! Limit yourself to 10–15 almonds per day.

Yogurt. Heavy, cold, and mucus-forming yogurt can be quite problematic for digestion. Good-quality dairy is not that easy to come by, and most yogurts available in stores are from unhappy and unhealthy cows. The word "Greek" on a yogurt container doesn't mean it is much better. It can still be filled with hormones, antibiotics, and hard-to-digest additives. If you love yogurt, always get organic and as fresh as possible. Unpasteurized goat and sheep's yogurt can be a better choice. Add some honey and cinnamon and serve at room temperature, not cold. The warming qualities of honey and cinnamon will help to counterbalance the yogurt's dampness.

Kale chips. Oh, how sorry I am to put kale chips on a no-no list. But remember this, the value of the item is not what is measured just by what the nutrition label lists; it is measured by what your body can assimilate from it and how much energy it will take to digest it. Kale, which is from the cabbage family, has a tendency to give gas to weak bellies. Dry chips of an already hard-on-the-stomach product will only make it worse. The toppings of nuts, spices, and protein powders turn kale chips into a gas-producing, constipating crunch. Have kale in stews, soups, or well-massaged salads instead.

Some other "healthy foods" that can aggravate digestion and lead to bloating and irregularity are crackers, granolas, dried fruits, protein bars, rice cakes, bottled juices, popcorn, chocolate (even the dark kind), whole-wheat bread, trail mix, pretzels, nondairy ice cream, bran muffins, jicama, and many more.

HAPPY BELLY SNACKS

In traditional ayurveda, there is no concept of "snacks." Ayurveda advises three balanced meals a day to allow for efficient digestion and absorption. The modern concept of grazing or eating five small meals a day would be rejected in ayurveda due to the potential negative effects on digestion. One of the main reasons that ayurveda doesn't recommend snacking is the time that it takes for each meal to digest. Depending on the ingredients and their combination, food can take anywhere from three to 12 hours to digest (refer to the *Food Transit Times* table in the color insert.) If you eat something before a previous meal is digested, you are prolonging the required digestion time and asking for bloating due to purification and fermentation.

There are no scientific studies that show that our metabolism actually speeds up when we eat every two hours. Unless you are a weightlifting professional or can make sure that you eat small enough portions of food that can be fully digested in two to three hours, it would be best to stick to larger meals and fewer snacks.

If you have blood sugar issues and you are making the transition to fewer snacks, you can experiment with these belly-friendly snacks. All of them are easy to digest for most people, won't cause bloating, and take a short amount of time to be digested.

Ten Belly-Friendly Snacks for Sensitive and Bloated Tummies

1. **Sprouted soaked and peeled almonds** (10–15). Chew slowly until liquid! Ayurveda recommends soaked and peeled almonds every day to build *ojas* (energy and the immune system).

2. **Warm apple sauce** with cinnamon, ghee, and ginger. Make your own or buy a "no sugar added" variety at the store.

3. **Stewed berries with a bit of coconut oil and cardamom**. Put a bowl of berries with coconut oil and cardamom in the oven for 10 minutes or microwave for one minute. (The microwave should not be used for daily cooking but only when you are in a rush.)

4. **Blueberries.** Many of us have an elevated amount of yeast in the body due to stress and poor diet. Sugars, even when they come from fruit, can create bloating in people with high yeast. Blueberries, because of their low sugar levels compared to other fruit, are less likely to upset the stomach even in someone recovering from yeast or candida.

5. **Avocado with pepper, lime, and good-quality salt.** Soft, nourishing, and rich, this fruit is surprisingly rich in protein and fiber. While quite heavy in texture, it is gentle on your stomach. According to ayurveda, avocado helps to build ojas

(energy and life force). If avocado is too difficult to digest, add lime, a pinch of salt, and cilantro. These ingredients will encourage the liver to release bile and effectively break down fats. Yummy!

6. **Date and coconut rolls with herbal ginger tea.** You can buy these in most health stores. Make sure no sugar is added and there are only two ingredients: dates and coconut.

7. **Pumpkin pie pudding.** Recipe: 1 cup of cooked pumpkin, 1 cup almond milk (add more if you want a smoothie instead of pudding), 1 banana, 2 packets of stevia, or 1.5 tablespoons honey or maple syrup (to taste), 2 teaspoons pumpkin pie spice blend, or 1.5 teaspoons cinnamon and 1/2 teaspoon ginger. Blend together.

8. **Roasted butternut squash with coconut oil, cinnamon and a few raisins.** Bake and keep in the fridge for a quick snack.

9. **Banana smoothie with lime, fresh ginger, and cardamom.** Bananas are smooth and mucilaginous for the mucus lining of the stomach. Lime, ginger, and cardamom help to digest banana. Blend one banana with a pinch of cardamom and fresh ginger and a squeeze of lime juice.

10. **Boiled or baked beets with a piece of raw goat milk cheese or sheep's milk ricotta and black pepper.** You can substitute baked squash or pumpkin for beets.

DAIRY DEBATE IN SHORT

Whether to go dairy-free or keep a dairy-friendly diet is a personal choice for everyone. It should be based on trial and observation of your body's reactions. Of course, if you choose to keep dairy in your diet there are a few things to keep in mind.

- Make it a priority to buy only organic, full-fat, unhomogenized milk. Milk we get in a plastic container at the store is very different, quality-wise, from fresh, raw milk straight from the cow. In India, many households in the countryside still get their milk brought to them by a milkman who walks from house to house with a cow and milks it right in front of you. Ultrapasteurized milk that lasts for weeks at the store might take just as long to be processed by overtaxed digestive systems, creating allergy-like symptoms.

- Learn to prepare your milk. Preparation methods for dairy products can be a huge determinant to whether your body can digest them and benefit from them. According to the science of ayurveda, there are ways to turn milk into a nectar, or, conversely, make it toxic to the body.

Here are three ways to have dairy that ayurveda lists as the easiest to digest and the most beneficial to the body.

- **Warm spiced milk.** Heating the milk makes it much easier for human consumption, and it reduces mucus, making it lighter to digest. Boil milk for five to ten minutes with cardamon, a cinnamon stick, and a few pinches of ginger.

- **Cumin lassi** (buttermilk). A lassi is plain yogurt and water, usually blended with cumin, lime, and pepper and used as a postmeal digestive. Get your recipe here: www. spinachanyoga.com/recipes.

- **Ghee.** In ayurveda, clarified butter, or ghee, is believed to be the best nutritional tonic for human beings. It is heat resistant and suitable for cooking. If prepared correctly, it does not have milk solids, and people with dairy intolerance can digest it well. It adds a rich buttery taste to oatmeal and an amazing flavor to sautéed vegetables. You can buy it at any organic health-food store, an Indian grocery, or you can make it yourself.

- **Soft mild cheese such as paneer and ricotta.** Make sure that they are fresh and made from the best quality milk you can get. Have mild cheeses with some black pepper and a generous serving of vegetables such as broccoli rabe, arugula, or kale. Avoid mixing with beans, yeasted wheat bread, and fruits.

On the other hand, in ayurveda, **cold milk or fruit-flavored yogurts are considered poisonous and mucus-forming**. Yogurt with fruit is another combination that ayurveda strictly forbids, as it is difficult to digest. Cream, hard, aged cheeses, or fat-reduced dairy options are considered too heavy and unsuitable for daily consumption. Ayurvedic physicians also advise against mixing dairy with acidic fruit, fish, or meat. Basically, if you have a weak stomach, consume dairy products separately from other foods.

FOODS AND THEIR PERSONALITIES

When we eat food, we take on the qualities of what we eat. Foods have personalities, and they change our personality to conform to theirs. Certain foods have very strong personalities and can significantly change the blood chemistry of a human being. Consuming such strong food on a regular basis takes you away from the real you. You are not 100 percent you anymore; you are *you*+coffee, or *you*+sugar.

Food affects not only your physical state but also your emotional state. Some foods will make you feel grounded, and others will evoke creativity and lightness. When you choose what goes on your plate, you can choose not only based on how you want your stomach to feel but also how you want to feel mentally and emotionally.

Food, according to ayurveda, is either *sattvic, rajasic, or tamasic,* according to its character and effect upon the body and the mind. The more we eat of a certain food, the more we take on the same qualities. Light, fresh, juicy vegetables create a happy, inspired person with a light, energetic body. Heavy, mucus-forming cakes and processed frozen TV dinners will more likely create a sluggish, dull, depressed person.

You don't need to learn the book on food energies by heart to know what and when to eat. It is more about being willing to pay attention to your body's response to food and allowing yourself to remember. You already know all this information, just as a dog knows when to chew on some grass when it needs to. Nobody told the dog to do it. He had that knowledge inside from generations ago. You do too. It is a matter of letting that wisdom come through and trusting it.

When you start cleaning out your diet from hard-to-digest foods and substituting lighter and easier foods, you are more likely to notice an emotional shift, as well. Your mind will be clearer, more inspired, and sharper. There might be some old emotions that show up and will need to be processed. Being kind, compassionate, and mindful during these shifts will help you to navigate them better.

Ayurveda classifies foods according to their effect on our body and mind. Understanding foods' properties can help you build a diet that creates a state of mind that you would like to experience and avoid emotions that you find unpleasant.

Here is how ayurveda classifies food and its effects on our emotions:

Sattvic food. Sattvic food is always fresh and simple. It is light, nourishing, sweet, and tasty. It increases the energy, creates a clear mind and supports cheerfulness, serenity, and mental clarity. Sattvic food is highly conducive to good health and happiness.

Sattvic food includes fresh ripe fruits, soaked nuts and seeds, dates, mung (tiny yellow lentils) sprouts, root vegetables such as sweet potatoes, easily digestible grains such as oats and rice (white), fresh organic dairy such as butter, ghee (clarified butter), and milk (if you can find unhomogenized organic milk and digest it well). Examples of sattvic foods are mango, figs, sprouted mung beans, land and sea vegetables, nut and seed milk, and herbal teas. The spices commonly used in sattvic cooking are turmeric, ginger, cinnamon, coriander, fennel, and cardamom.

The sattvic way of eating is not rushed; it is mindful, done in good company, or in silence.

The sattvic personality: people who follow the sattvic way of eating are known to be clear-minded, balanced, and spiritually aware.[41] In my personal experience, I find that eating a predominantly sattvic diet helps in meditation and yoga practice and helps to avoid feelings of irritation, anger, or fatigue. However, it also makes people very sensitive to their surroundings and might not be the easiest diet to maintain when living in a large city.

Rajasic food. This is food that is fresh but heavy and stimulating. It includes nonvegetarian food such as fresh organic chicken; cage-free eggs; wild fish; all lentils (not sprouted); hot spices, such as chilies and peppers; nightshades, such as tomatoes; and pungent vegetables, such onion and garlic. The rajasic diet is also cooked fresh and is nutritious. It may contain a little more oil and spices compared to sattvic food. It benefits those who believe in action, ambition, and an active social life, in other words, it benefits most of us living in the modern world.

Rajasic foods include lemon, tea, and organic coffee. Rajasic way of eating is to consume food very quickly.

The rajasic personality: Rajasic foods create people with strong emotions, desires, goals, and ambitions. People who eat a predominantly rajastic diet are in control of their lives. They are go-getters and know how to enjoy life.

Personally, I find that I feel good eating a predominantly sattvic diet with some rajasic foods in it.

Tamasic foods. These foods include foods that are overcooked, stale, and processed: foods made from refined flour, pastries, pizzas, burgers, processed chocolate, soft drinks, white bread, canned and preserved foods — such as jams — pickles, fermented foods, fried foods, sweets made from sugar, ice creams, and puddings. All overly spicy, salty, sweet, and fatty foods form part of the tamasic diet.

Overeating or eating while upset and angry is tamasic. It creates dullness of mind, fatigue, and lack of enthusiasm.

The tamasic personality: Tamasic foods bring about stagnation leading to degeneration of health. According to ayurveda, someone who follows a predominantly tamasic diet may suffer from intense mood swings, insecurity, desires, and cravings, and is unable to deal with others in a balanced way. Their nervous systems and hearts do not function optimally, and such individuals age quickly, according to ayurveda. The tamasic diet can also create a favorable environment for degenerative diseases, cancers, diabetes, arthritis, and chronic fatigue.

VEGAN, VEGETARIAN, PALEO, OR CARNIVORE?

This question often comes up when I work with people in groups or one-on-one. What should I be? What diet should I follow?

You can be an unhealthy vegetarian who eats fast food, fries, and Oreo cookies, and drinks processed sodas, just as much as you can be a meat eater who lives on processed turkey slices, factory eggs, and canned soups. You can also be a balanced, mindful vegetarian who eats whole grains, raw dairy, and lots of seasonal vegetables. Or you can be a healthy meat eater, who eats meat one to two times a week, opts for wild-caught fish, cage-free eggs, and consumes lots of fresh vegetables, legumes, and fruit.

Labeling yourself this or that won't automatically make you healthy. Any diet should be mindful. So I encourage you not to squeeze into any labels. Be a person who listens to the body more than magazine covers and who eats whole foods.

Many things have a strong effect on our body without us fully understanding how they work. For example, when a doctor gives you a pill, you might not know the way it works on a chemical level, but you feel that it definitely affects you. The same thing happens with many foods and practices. Noticing the effect may take longer and usually is determined by how attentive and sensitive to the internal shifts you are, but they do definitely happen.

For example, there are lots of books on the vegan raw way of eating. Lots of people claim incredible benefits from this diet and way of living. I love vegan and raw foods. My meals are often vegan and in the summer can be predominantly raw. But on an intuitive level, I know that I wouldn't feel good at this stage of my life on a fully raw vegan diet. I need more grounding. Living in a big city, I need warmth during cold weather. I need more density when my emotions run wild.

However cheesy it might sound, when choosing your own diet, you have to listen to your body. Your body knows best. It also changes all the time, so your needs will change too. An irritated, inflamed gut might feel better with lean protein than legumes and grains that might be too coarse. But once you heal and your digestion is stronger, you might feel drawn to more vegetables, raw foods, and fruits.

In the beginning, listening to your body's wisdom or advice is not easy. There is a lot of white noise in the form of what other people are saying, articles and books you've read, common beliefs, and commercials. To hear what your body is saying, all of this noise needs to go to the background. The easiest way to do this is to imagine that you don't know a thing about food and base your decisions only on *how you feel.*

This is when a detailed food log comes in very handy. It helps to speed up the learning process. It can help you notice trends that come with eating certain foods. You will notice that certain foods trigger positive or negative emotions, a different state of mind, a different level of energy. If we don't pay attention to these shifts, we will never learn and will always have to rely on someone to tell us what to eat.

INDIVIDUALIZATION

Each human being is unique and needs a unique approach to life and food to feel balanced and thriving. There are many different diets and approaches to nutrition that can create a thriving healthy human being. There have been tribes all over the world eating different traditional diets and living healthily. One of the common threads of most healthy diets is *real unprocessed* food, very limited sugar, and lots of physical movement in the fresh air. Our body is very adaptable and is meant to thrive under different conditions.

Since everyone is different and has different needs, no whole food, plant, or herb can be classified as generally "good" or "bad." Each one can be a medicine or a poison depending on the situation. Processed food doesn't count. One of my favorite teachers, Dr. Claudia Welch, says, "We learn in ayurveda that there are no universally and inherently 'good' foods or 'bad' foods. The old saying, 'one man's meat is another man's poison' finds acceptance in ayurvedic philosophy. Ayurvedic classics teach us that there is no substance on earth that cannot act as a medicine in certain situations. We simply must understand the qualities of the substance and the person, in order to understand how it is likely to affect them."

Chapters 22 and 23 also talk about individualization, so make sure you read them as well.

We will discuss in more detail what foods and lifestyle changes work for someone with bloating, constipation, or acid reflux in the fourth part of the book, "Resolving Specific Issues."

HERBAL TEAS TO SOOTHE INDIGESTION AND BLOATING

In ayurveda, spices are regarded as medicine. Each spice has its medicinal properties and can enhance not only the flavor of food but its healing powers. It is believed that spices improve digestion by stimulating our digestive fire, which in Western terms can mean the production of enzymes and improving circulation. Adding a little bit of spice to your food is similar to taking the currently popular digestive enzymes. You can use spices in food or in teas. There are lots of books on spices and their healing powers, but a few of these teas will get you started.

You can make functional teas to ease the symptoms of indigestion, such as gas, bloating, pain and diarrhea, or constipation. These recipes can be made from spices usually found in your kitchen cabinet or easily found at your local grocery. Make sure to buy fresh spices and avoid old, stale spices, or those not stored in an air-tight container.

Happy Belly indigestion tea. This simple tea works well for the bloated belly. It can be taken one to two times per day before lunch and dinner. It is best to sip this tea a half hour before meals. Put 1/2 teaspoon each of coriander seeds, cumin seeds, and fennel seeds in four cups of water. Bring to a boil, let steep, strain, and drink. In the summer, add fresh mint and lime juice. Coriander, cumin, and fennel tea is cooling and soothing for the mind, digestion, and urinary tract. These three kitchen spices are balancing for all seasons and body types.

Sexy and cool. Dried rose petals, cardamom pods, fennel seeds and fresh ginger. Rose petals are considered cooling in ayurveda. Cardamom is considered an excellent digestive, especially beneficial for bloating and intestinal gas.[42] Ginger is a zesty spice useful in aiding digestion, promoting appetite, and helping with occasional stomach discomfort. Fennel is also cooling and exceptionally beneficial for IBS, bloating, and gas. For a one-liter pot, boil water and pour it over three tablespoons of dried rose petals, five to six cardamom pods, three tablespoons of fennel, and one inch of crushed ginger root. Let it steep covered for five to ten minutes and enjoy throughout the day plain or with lime.

Coriander tea. This tea soothes and heals the entire digestive tract. Bring to a boil one teaspoon of coriander in one cup of water. Steep for five to ten minutes. Strain and drink.

Ginger tea. Ginger tea is simple yet very effective in awakening a sluggish digestion in the morning. Ginger is warming and can help to reduce mucus and stimulate the digestive tract. Due to this stimulating action on the digestion, it is also the perfect drink to be taken either before you eat a meal or half an hour afterward. Cut one inch of fresh ginger to one liter of water. Bring to the boil and simmer for at least five minutes. Add lime and/or honey. Strain into a mug and enjoy!

Peppermint tea. Peppermint tea is extremely useful for indigestion, GI cramps, and relieving IBS pain and gut spasms. Peppermint has an antispasmodic action, with a calming effect on the muscles of the stomach, intestinal tract, and uterus.[43] It also has powerful analgesic (pain-killing) properties. You can use fresh mint leaves or loose-leaf peppermint tea.

Spicy limeade. To stimulate toxin release, try hot water with a pinch of cayenne, one-quarter lime, one teaspoon honey, and a few drops of apple cider vinegar. This ayurvedic blend will boost fat digestion and metabolism, according to the ayurvedic practicioner John Immel, the founder of Joyful Belly. A strong sour taste encourages the free flow of bile from your liver and gall bladder to your gut. This spicy drink restores energy and vitality by helping the body digest high-fat foods. Vinegar and cayenne add an intense metabolic spark that improves energy and enthusiasm. Together with warm water, they strongly stimulate digestion and clear mucus accumulations from the stomach. This has the effect of improving circulation and revving up metabolism. Drink only once a day. This drink is heating, so it would be good for people who are heavy and feel sluggish. It is not recommended for people with high acidity, skin inflammation, rashes, or rapid metabolism.

TRADITIONAL AYURVEDIC REMEDIES

Lemon ginger salt remedy. This remedy resets and rekindles the digestive fire. It stimulates the digestive juices and thereby promotes better digestion. The lemon ginger salt remedy is particularly beneficial for the person who experiences bloating or indigestion due to overeating, munching, or eating late at night. To prepare this remedy, grate some fresh ginger, add a small amount of fresh lemon juice, and add a pinch or two of salt. Eat a few pinches of this mixture one half hour prior to lunch and dinner each day.

Ayurvedic stomach-gas relief recipe. This recipe works especially well for the bloating which happens within the first few bites of a meal at the top of the stomach. Relief should occur within minutes. Mix one-eighth of a teaspoon of powdered (not fresh) ginger with one teaspoon of honey. Mix with hot water. The most effective way to take this remedy is to chew the mixture and then drink hot water.

SPICES TO BUY

Ginger: It has a powerful carminative effect—meaning that it aids in the prevention of flatulence. It can also help cleanse and heal the digestive tract. It can help to relieve muscle cramping.

Coriander: Coriander is one of the best herbs for supporting digestion without aggravating pitta. It enkindles the digestive fire while simultaneously cooling and soothing the GI tract. It helps to clear the digestive tract of trapped gas after a meal. Coriander seed oil will stimulate the production of gastric juices, and therefore help to stimulate appetite. It has been used in India for its anti-inflammatory properties.

Fennel: The United States once listed fennel as an official drug to be used for digestive problems, and the herb is still used daily as an after-dinner digestive aid from Spain to India to Italy. Fennel has antispasmodic properties, and it stimulates the production of gastric juices. It's useful for gastrointestinal and menstrual cramps, heartburn, diarrhea, colic, stomachaches, and indigestion.

Cumin: Cumin is one of the best herbs for supporting healthy digestion without aggravating pitta. A common household spice, its Sanskrit name literally means "promoting digestion." In addition to providing flavor to food, Cumin kindles the digestive fire, promotes healthy absorption, and eliminates natural toxins in the GI tract. The seeds are often chewed after meals and are especially useful for calming excess vata in the lower abdomen and in promoting a comfortable postdining experience.

Cinnamon: Soothes digestive discomfort, improves digestive capacity, boosts immunity, and balances blood sugar.

TRUTH ABOUT EXERCISE AND DIGESTION

If you have ever researched or asked your doctor about ways to improve your digestion, most likely you have heard that you should exercise on a regular basis. Exercise improves blood circulation, lymphatic drainage, and in general helps things to move along.

However, what I noticed in the process of studying digestion and working with people on improving it is that not all exercise has the same effect. Some exercises will actually help counteract bloating and constipation, while others can foster them!

It might sound pretty crazy, but certain exercise habits can make elimination less regular and as a result create digestive problems. I have experienced it myself and seen it in many other women.

Below, I will share a few of my observations on bad exercise habits and offer ways to avoid negative effects on the intricate digestive balance.

The following exercise habits are not conducive to a happy belly:

- **Not breathing properly while exercising.** A lot of instructors will encourage people to hold their stomach in almost all the time. While core engagement can help stabilization and protect the spine, not letting the diaphragm come down during the breath is not a good habit. When we breathe fully, our stomach should naturally extend to allow the diaphragm to move down. Full breath = more oxygen in the blood = more energy to exercise and better digestion. When we hold the stomach in – this turns into a habit even outside the yoga or Pilates class – it can negatively impact digestion. A soothing, massaging effect of deep abdominal breathing and a relaxed stomach make a huge difference in the functioning of the digestive and reproductive systems. Check in with yourself to make sure that you are not holding your breath when working hard and that each breath is complete. You should feel your abdominal area slightly expanding when you inhale.

- **Doing core exercises without stretching afterwards.** In general, crunches, sit-ups, side planks, and twists are great for digestion. They can help to improve circulation to the organs in the abdominal area and stimulate regularity. However, doing only contraction-type movements without creating extension through stretching afterward can leave all the muscles around your digestive system tight. When things are tight, there is not enough space for movement, so things (your waste) will get stuck. Make sure to always stretch and balance out the contractions with extensions. Cat/cow or a cobra pose are great stretches to try after a core-toning routine.

- **Dehydration.** It hurts me to watch people working on cardio machines or in intense classes without water. When exercise raises your body temperature and you are sweating buckets, your body is losing precious water. Considering that most people are dehydrated to begin with, extra water loss is not a welcome change in the body. When dehydrated, our body draws water from the colon to provide enough hydration for other organs, such as the heart and liver. If too much water from the stool and colon is reabsorbed back into the body, you get constipated. Fortunately, this problem is pretty easy to solve. Before working out, make your own rehydrating drink with lemon, some sea salt, and honey, or just sip on room-temperature water with electrolytes but no sugar.

On the other hand, some exercises are incredibly helpful when it comes to improving elimination and preventing bloating.

My favorite happy belly exercises are:

- **Yoga.** It is a multifunctional tool. It helps to resolve many issues that get in the way of connecting to your true self, including feeling constipated or bloated. It's easier to meditate, to feel at peace, and to feel at home living in a body that is free of waste. You can adapt your yoga practice to address the issue of digestion just the same way you adjust your diet to address your needs. Compression/ extension of the abdomen, such as in a cat/cow or down-dog into up-dog sequence, side stretching such as an extended side angle and triangle, and backbends are all very helpful. If you want to learn all the yoga tricks for improving digestion, watch my *Yoga for Digestion* videos on www.spinachandyoga.com/videos.

- **Dancing and shaking your hips.** Belly dancing and Latin- inspired dancing are great ways to get things moving! Dancing helps to move muscles of the abdominal and pelvic region, which massages deeper internal organs. The result is better intestine and colon health. Remember, though, don't eat for at least an hour or two before you dance. Having food content in the stomach while shaking your hips can make you nauseous.

- **Rebounder/trampoline.** This one is addictive! Rebounding stimulates the circulation of lymphatic fluid, the body's waste disposal mechanism, providing direct support to your immune and digestive system. For me, any exercise has to feel good and be fun, and rebounding is both. It is a great cardioendurance-toning workout. I have my rebounder sitting in the living room and I often take breaks from work to jump for a few minutes.

- **Brisk walking.** Walking is amazing. You get outside, breathe fresh air, get vitamin D, and get your body moving. The gentle bouncing movement of walking helps to improve circulation and digestion, as well. So get outside and go for a walk.

EXERCISE, STRESS, AND SELF-ABUSE

Most of us do not realize that the high-intensity exercise that is so loved by many can be a stressor. Our body responds to exercise as an emergency. The fight-or-flight nervous system gets activated, and this emergency response during each workout produces stress-fighting, degenerative hormones. Considering that most big-city dwellers have drained adrenal glands and don't have time to stretch after a workout to calm down the nervous system, extreme workouts, over time, can do more harm than good. As you remember, stress and digestion are very closely connected. Overly depleting exercise for the type A women who run on caffeine is another factor that can contribute to an inflamed gut.

Women in general are very disconnected from their bodies, especially the stomach and pelvic area. If you want your life to flow easily and effortlessly, you need to learn what it feels like in the body to move with pleasure and ease. You need to reconnect to your body and feel it. It means not doing things based on what someone thinks is right but listening to your body and letting it decide what's right for today.

It is scary to let go of the five-times-a-week cardio routine. You might be afraid that you will gain weight, that your body will turn flabby, and you will move away even further from your dream body. I felt the same. It took a pretty strong signal on the part of my body to slow down and start listening. Dr. Claudia Welch's book *Balance Your Hormones, Balance Your Life* helped me to take the leap of faith—faith in the idea that my body knows better than any fitness expert.

I started by cutting down my elliptical workouts and doing a bit more yoga in the morning. In just a couple of days my body felt a lot more energized and rested and my stomach felt at ease and flat. I felt more in the flow, more feminine, more connected, and there was a deeper degree of trust between my body and me.

Belly dancing, S factor, yoga, abdominal breathing, and massage help to get the connection back. It does make one feel a lot more in tune, feminine, and sexual, besides improving digestion.

It's important to mention here that I'm not encouraging you to stop exercising. Instead, I invite you to find a type of movement that makes you feel the way you want to feel. If you want to feel more feminine, look for that in your exercise routine; if you want more strength, look for that. Be very clear on what you want to experience in your body as a final goal.

Think of exercise as an act of self-love. We need movement that is nourishing, fun, playful, not draining, and not aggravating to digestion but instead gets the lymphatic system and the circulation going. If it doesn't make you smile, it is not the best thing for you right now.

Exercise is a tool, not a goal of its own, unless you are a professional. Exercise is a tool that helps to create an optimal, healthy body that allows you to enjoy life and never feel constricted by physical discomforts.

Good reasons to exercise are to keep your heart healthy, to improve circulation, to improve and enkindle digestive fire, to feel connected to your body, to get lymph moving, and to have fun.

Bad reasons to exercise are to punish yourself for overeating, to change the body parts that you hate, to become like an actress or model, or because somebody told you to do it.

Keep exercise mindful and focused. Exercise should be aligned to your ideal image of self. This is the time to connect to that image.

For specific belly-friendly yoga routines, go here: www. spinachandyoga.com/videos.

chapter 26

SUPPLEMENTS

Under the guidance of Dana James, a certified nutritionist and the founder of Food Coach NYC, who has a lot of experience working with food sensitivities and also has done careful research on the subject, I created a list of supplements that you can discuss with your doctor to help with GI symptoms.

Before jumping to pills, I would start by experimenting with diet, herbal teas, and habits around food. However, when the inflammation is persistent and the symptoms are not going away, you can use supplements to help your body in healing.

Some supplements and herbs to consider (for a full list and the best brands, check out the Happy Belly online store at www. spinachandyoga.com/HappyBellyShop).

- Fennel, ginger teas, especially Gaia herbs digestion teas to combat bloating and indigestion.

- Triphala pills and powder—have a mild detoxifying and tonifying effect.

- Aloe vera gel and juice. Sugar-free aloe vera juice can help restore GI integrity and decrease inflammation. Lily of the Desert is a great brand.

- Glutamine is an amino acid that helps restore gut barrier function. Take five grams of glutamine powder in the morning and evening. This can be combined with herbs such as slippery elm, chamomile, marshmallow, licorice, and coptis root which all help to regenerate the lining of the GI tract. Some people are very sensitive to herbs, so if you don't respond well to them, simply take straight glutamine powder.

- Peppermint oil and/or tea.

- Calcium/magnesium citrate. It promotes stress-reduction and regularity. CALM is a good brand.

- Chlorophyll and E3LIVE. They help to reduce inflammation, reduce acidity, and are easily absorbable minerals.

- Probiotics and prebiotics are two of the most important supplements you can take to help restore healthy digestion. Probiotics provide live strains of friendly bacteria that are crucial for digestive, immune, and neurological health. Prebiotics ensure that your friendly flora is provided with a nourishing environment in which they can thrive. Upon waking, take a 12-strain probiotic with 50 billion IU and saccharomyces boulardii. The probiotics will help to repopulate the gut with microflora to reduce the proliferation of pathogenic microbes, while the saccharomyces boulardii will help create SIgA, which helps the gut lining fight off invading microbes.

- Zinc is an important nutrient for digestive health. It also plays critical roles in hormone regulation, immune health, and neurological function.

- Fish oils reduce inflammation and help heal GI tract lining, improve nutrient absorption, balance hormones, improve neurological function, and boost immunity.

- Protolytic enzymes increase digestive capacity and nutrient absorption, boost immunity, and increase vital energy.

- B12 helps heal the lining of the GI tract.

- Slippery elm bark tea coats the digestive tract, making it less likely to leak molecules into the blood.

part 4

RESOLVING
SPECIFIC ISSUES

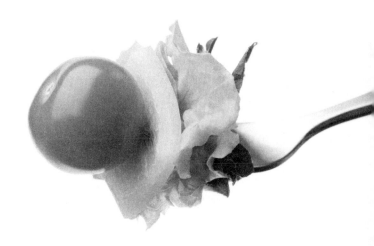

chapter 27

BLOATING AND GAS CURE

Nobody likes the feeling of a bloated stomach. Unfortunately, most women are familiar with the unpleasant feeling of a bloated belly. It feels as if you have a balloon in your stomach that's weighing you down, making you feel heavy, and not sexy at all! This usually happens right when you need to get dressed to go out for dinner or are planning a fun night on the town with your girlfriends. Bloating doesn't help with the romantic part of your life either. What is more of a "mood killer" than feeling as if you swallowed a basketball?

Bloating is not only detrimental to our self-confidence but can also have negative effects on your health. Bloating usually occurs as a result of too much fermentation in the digestive tract. It can happen due to stress, food sensitivity, lack of necessary enzymes, uncoordinated peristalsis, or as a reaction to too much fiber. According to ayurveda, bloating is a sign of a weak digestive fire.

When we have too much gas forming internally, it could mean that the food is staying longer in the digestive tract than it should so the bacteria has more time to ferment the leftovers in the intestines.

This excessive fermentation can irritate the wall of the intestines, making them thinner and even leading to leaky gut.

The byproducts of fermentation are toxins that are absorbed into the blood and over time can weaken liver and kidneys. According to ayurveda, a strong body odor is one of the signs of excessive fermentation and toxins in the blood. It can also weaken the immune system and give you acne. Our nervous system is very sensitive to chemical changes in the blood. Toxins in the blood lead to emotional disturbances, lack of clear thinking, and anxiety.

Besides making you feel more attractive and comfortable in your body, reducing bloating will reduce your body's toxic burden. It will also improve nutrient absorption since most of that happens in the intestines.

I used to experience bloating quite a bit before introducing ayurveda and conscious eating into my daily life. Bloating is mostly a result of improper eating habits such as eating in a rush without properly chewing food, overeating, drinking cold water, and eating when stressed. Food sensitivities and a leaky gut are often a result of bad eating habits, overabundance of hard-to-digest foods, and stress. However, once you develop food sensitivities and a leaky gut, a vicious cycle begins. The more irritated your intestines are, the more likely you are to experience bloating and gas, among other symptoms. And if this is not addressed, more and more foods will lead to these unpleasant reactions.

According to ayurveda, bloating and gas can be triggered by an excessive amount of cold and hard-to-digest foods. Cabbage, ice, and beans are good examples. Raw food is more difficult to digest than cooked foods for someone with a weak digestion. Ice cream and anything with ice reduces the supply of blood and is also more likely to trigger the symptoms. Underchewing food makes it harder to digest. Throwing big pieces of food into your stomach requires a lot more work to be done internally. Sometimes we forget that there are no teeth in your stomach! Drink your food and chew your liquids. Poor food combination, especially mixing dairy and fruit with anything else, can cause bloating in many people.

Some people are more subject to bloating due to hormonal imbalances or weakened digestion after years of improper food combining and relying on hard-to-digest foods such as wheat. The good thing is that bloating is preventable and your intestines can heal like any other muscle.

I still remember that unpleasant feeling of a full belly even after a small meal, and it makes me happy that I found ways to prevent it. Now that I've found a solution for myself, I want to share what works for me and, hopefully, some of you will find these suggestions useful as well.

Conscious eating and including lots of easy-to-digest foods are two of the main components for preventing bloating. If you are aware of how your stomach feels, how hungry you are, and the effects that foods have on your body, you will be able to adapt your eating habits accordingly. I believe that people who are truly conscious and follow their intuition rarely experience digestive unease.

PREVENT BLOATING

It is best to prevent bloating, instead of trying to address the issue when it is already there. It is a lot easier and will save you the trouble of experiencing this pretty unpleasant feeling. So the suggestion list will start with prevention strategies.

1. **Eat only when truly hungry.** Try to avoid emotional eating and overeating. Go back to page 84 for more tips on overcoming emotional eating.

2. **Allow your previous meal to fully digest before eating the next meal.** That means waiting at least three hours between meals.

3. **While eating, chew well and don't talk while chewing.** If you are eating with others, put your fork down in between bites and let the flavor and the experience of food be your only focus. DON'T EAT and TALK at the same time. Better yet, meet friends for walks or for tea and keep social eating to a minimum until your gut is healthy and strong. See "Mindful Eating 101" on page 184.

4. **Be careful with your fiber:** Coarse or poorly chewed fiber will delay passage through the digestive system and slow down the rate at which the food is digested and absorbed. So if you don't chew a slice of bread or a piece of potato properly, you are leaving a lot more work for your stomach and digestion will take longer. One of the things that is important to keep in mind here is that the longer carbohydrate food stays in your intestines, the more time bacteria has to ferment it. Fermentation can lead to gas and bloating.

5. **Follow general food combining rules** (see color insert).

6. **Eat easy-to-digest meals when in a rush, stressed, or anxious.** Focus on soupy, warm, monomeals such as kitchari,

soups, smoothies, and sautéed vegetables. Follow the Happy Belly meal plan as outlined in the color insert.

7. **Eat fruit at least 20–30 minutes before meals.** Don't eat fruit after a meal. It will be gas forming and produce bloating.

8. **Try chewing on a slice of ginger with lime juice** or lemon 20 minutes before a meal.

9. **Use digestion-stimulating spices when making your food.** Try black pepper, ginger, cumin, coriander, cardamom, fennel, and asafoetida for beans.

10. **Try adding enzymes**, especially to heavy meals.

11. **Regularly take probiotics**, especially if you have been on antibiotics recently.

12. **Pay attention to how your body reacts to dairy and flour products.** If you feel bloated after them, you might have to cut down. It will be a lot easier to convince yourself to do it once you feel a direct correlation between eating those products and a bloated stomach. If you are not willing to take a weeklong break from dairy and flour, then opt for a food sensitivity test such as ALCAT to find out if you have a problem.

13. **Drink a glass of warm or room temperature water with lime to hydrate 30 minutes before eating.**

14. **Don't drink anything cold while eating.** Preferably, limit cold foods as well. Fruits should be room temperature, not

straight from the fridge. If you can't live without your ice cream (dairy or nondairy), have some ginger tea afterward.

15. Avoid drinking anything 30 minutes after the meal. It will dilute digestive juices and will make it harder to digest food.

16. Reduce SALT. The easiest way to do that is to start cooking your own meals. Restaurant meals are often overly salty.

17. Eliminate caffeine and alcohol if you have a leaky gut or inflammation.

18. Try aromatherapy. Bloating is more likely to appear if you are anxious, stressed, or worried. Try peppermint, orange, rose, cinnamon, or basil essential oils. You can also just get a stress-relieving or balancing essential oil mix at most health food stores.

19. Learn Agnisar Kriya. Do it every morning before a meal and after having a glass of warm water with lemon. I have been doing it for years and besides promoting strong abs and a flat stomach, it is great for all digestion-related issues. Watch the video tutorial at www. spinachandyoga.com/videos.

20. Keep a food journal to track which foods or which food combinations trigger the symptoms. You can download a Food Log at www.spinachandyoga.com/resources.

21. Do a daily visualization focusing on your stomach being flat, and your digestion strong and regular. Download a guided visualization at www.spinachandyoga.com/resources.

IF YOU FEEL BLOATED, TRY THESE REMEDIES

1. **Chew on a few fennel seeds or sip a hot fennel and ginger tea**. Prepare fennel tea by crushing one teaspoon of fennel seed and adding it to one cup of water in a pot. Bring the water to a boil, and cover and steep it for 10 to 15 minutes. Cool and strain. A traditional dose of fennel tea is about two to three cups daily. If you are at a restaurant or don't have fennel seeds, opt for a mint/peppermint tea. It is also soothing to the digestive tract. You can also carry tea bags in your bag. For a list of my favorite tummy teas, go to www.spinachandyoga.com/HappyBellyShop.

2. **Do five minutes of deep abdominal breathing**. Don't hold your stomach in.

3. **Lay on your left side and breathe deeply.**

4. **Go for a brisk walk for 30 minutes**. I like doing a few jumping jacks or twists. It helps to increase blood circulation (since your heart will be beating faster) and to release gas.

5. **Do a child's pose, wind-relieving pose, seated twists,** poses that create extension and contraction of the abdomen such as cat/cow.

6. **Apply a warm compress on the lower part of the stomach or take a warm bath** to improve circulation and counteract muscle contraction that might be causing bloating.

This list is long and might seem overwhelming in the beginning, but different things work for different people. Try a few of the above tips and listen to your body's feedback. Soon you will be able to find a few antibloating tricks that work for your unique body. Experiment and learn!

BEANS AND LENTILS WITHOUT GAS

There is a lot of controversy around the effect of beans and lentils on our digestive system.

Historically, legumes have played a key role in the diet of many cultures. They are the cheapest source of protein and can be very delicious if cooked properly. In the Western world most of the population looks down on legumes. What got us so scared? And why does our stomach react to legumes with bloating and gas?

Galactomannans (polymers) are a type of fiber present in legumes and some manufactured foods such as guar gum and locust bean gum, which are often used as thickening agents. These water-soluble and often viscous polysaccharides (large complex sugars) also remain undigested in the small intestine, and can exert important effects on digestive physiology.

A great article from the Weston A. Price Foundation[44] states: "When consumed, oligosaccharides (a type of fiber) reach the lower intestine largely intact, and in the presence of anaerobic bacteria, ferment and produce carbon dioxide and methane gases, as well as a good deal of discomfort."

Beans cause gas because they contain saponins to protect themselves against insects. Saponins form the sudsy foam on the surface of a cooking pot of beans. They prevent protein digestion, resulting in fermentation and gas.

Most people don't know how to cook with grains and legumes to neutralize their gas-producing, gut-irritating qualities. Most beans and lentils in restaurants are undercooked or cooked improperly and because of that are more likely to trigger gas and bloating.

Traditionally, legumes are soaked for prolonged periods of time, cooked over several hours or even overnight on low heat and with digestion-stimulating spices.

How to Keep Legumes in Your Diet without Gas and Gut Irritation

Keep the dishes simple. No meat-beans-grains-bread-cheese-and-sour-cream combo unless you have a stomach of steel! Declutter your dishes and simplify! A great dish to try is mung bean soup or traditional dhal, such as in www.spinachandyoga.com/recipes.

Soak all legumes, grains, and nuts overnight to neutralize phytic acid. Change the water several times throughout the soaking process.

Add spices such as cumin, coriander, fennel, kombu seaweed, ginger, and hing.

Cook slowly and on low heat. A slow cooker is ideal. Eat small quantities of these foods and not every day.

Neutralizing Phytic Acid

LEGUME VARIETY	OPTIMAL WATER PH	SOAKING TIME	BEST SOAKING MEDIUM
Black beans	5.5	18–24 hours	Water with lemon juice, vinegar, or whey added
Lentils	5.0	10 hours	Water with lemon juice, vinegar, or whey added
Fava beans	4.0	10 hours	Water with lemon juice, vinegar, or whey added
Dried and split peas	7.0 to 7.5	10 hours	Plain soft water with pinch of baking soda
Brown, white & kidney beans	7.0	18–24 hours	Plain soft water

This table appeared in *Wise Traditions in Food, Farming and the Healing Arts*, the quarterly magazine of the Weston A. Price Foundation, Winter 2006.

chapter 28

······································

RESTORE REGULARITY

I t might be funny to talk about such personal stuff online or in a book, but if there is something that gets in the way of the optimal functioning of our body, I have to tell you about this. I just can't make myself shut up about digestion. It is crucial to our well-being, happiness, and ability to look good.

Americans spend over $725 million on laxatives each year. This is not accounting for endless fiber supplements, herbal colon cleanses, and other digestive aids. Getting Americans to poop is a booming billion-dollar industry! Looking at these numbers makes me think that I am surrounded by constipated people. And it always makes me sad.

Constipation, while not life-threatening in most cases, can be quite debilitating. Being constipated can lead to an array of problems: bad breath, weight gain, allergies, bloating, poor nutrient assimilation, fatigue, migraine, breakouts, heartburn, lower back pain, and, sadly, the list goes on. Unfortunately, many people have come to believe that going to the bathroom two to three times a week is normal. That is bad news since all the waste that is not eliminated is rotting inside and changes the blood chemistry in your body, allowing disease to set in. Practitioners of traditional Chinese medicine and ayurveda believe the Western pooping norm is abnormal. In ayurveda we believe that we should have a bowel movement every day. Skipping a day is not scary, but it is a sign that something is off.

To be diagnosed with constipation at the doctor's office you need to meet the following criteria, with two or more of the following criteria present for 12 or more weeks during the last 12 months.

- fewer than three stools per week.

- straining in 25 percent or more of defecations.

- lumpy or hard stools at least 25 percent of the time.

- sense of anorectal obstruction or blockage at least 25 percent of the time.

Most people never go to the doctor with such issues, and as a result, the issue is often not dealt with. People just learn to live with it and get used to the discomfort and side effects. In reality, this issue of irregularity is very common. When I was giving a talk at TED Talent Search in NYC on improving digestion, I asked the audience, "How many of you had a satisfying poop this morning?" I got a few hands, a few giggles, and lots of interested looks in the hopes of learning something that would help with the morning elimination habit.

The importance of healthy elimination in ayurveda is summarized by the phrase, "You are as healthy as your colon."

Digestion builds blood and feeds all our organs. To create good blood, we need good digestion.

- If fecal matter stays inside too long, food starts to rot and create toxins and waste products. Waste products can irritate the intestines. It can create a feeling of heaviness and bloating.

- Gray lusterless skin is usually a sign of chronic constipation (sign of toxins in the blood), along with lack of eye brightness, and a thick tongue coating.

- Toxins can create emotional disturbances and affect neurons and neurotransmitters.

- Constipation often leads to tight muscles.

- The immune system can be affected by chronic constipation.

- Joint pain (arthritis) and constipation are related.

You have about 20 feet (six meters) of small intestine. There are actually *three* parts to your small intestine. The first two are involved in breaking down food. The last part is where all the nutrients are absorbed. At this stage, it's all quite "liquidy" with all the gastric juices from your stomach and secretions from your pancreas. Next, undigested food and fiber move into the final five feet (1.5 meters) of the journey called the large intestine (or colon) where the excess water is reabsorbed into the body.

There are multiple causes for constipation including dehydration, too much dry food in the diet, food allergies or sensitivities, too many cold foods that constrict blood vessels, or just being cold in general (when you are cold you tighten up and constrict, versus letting things flow), stress, being in a rush especially in the morning, lack of fiber, bad bacteria in the gut, changes in the hormones, as before your period, and certain diseases and medications.

Sometimes constipation can be attributed to the nervous system. Tension can be created by feeling in a rush or not feeling comfortable in the bathroom, if not at home or by generally not feeling safe and feeling vulnerable. Historically, it was not the best time to go to the bathroom if you were not safe. When threatened in nature, we get ready to run or fight, not poop. A good way to know if you have this type of constipation is to compare your bowel habits when you are relaxed and not rushed to the days when you are tense, not at home, or under a lot of stress.

Being regular and bloat-free takes intimacy because you can't do it without truly getting to know your body. You also need to analyze your habits around food, diet, and lifestyle to see if you can find a physical or an emotional root cause behind irregularity. Once you know what the root cause is, it will be a lot easier to address it than trying things randomly in the hope of getting lucky.

If your diet is predominantly dry, full of astringent taste, and not enough liquid, trying to relax and meditate won't have as much of an effect as adding more hydration and moisture. If the reason is emotional tension, it should also be addressed with emotional work, not just a diet of soups and prunes.

How to Restore Regularity—General Tips

1. **Add it to your routine.** Yes, I know it sounds funny, but it is one of the most profound things you can try. It should be a part of your morning cleansing routine. In our crazy busy lives, a lot of things have to be scheduled in advance to get done. Going to the bathroom is no exception! Making it a habit is similar to training a puppy to go out at the same times each day. It takes some practice, but then it works like magic. We are creatures of habit, and our body thrives in a familiar routine. Even if you don't feel an urge to go to the bathroom right away, sit on the toilet and focus on breathing (no phone in your hands, though!). Over time, your body will connect the dots, appreciate your nonhurried effort, and start cooperating.

2. **Stop constant snacking.** Don't eat until the previous meal is digested. Do a quick check-in with your belly before and after eating. If you do snack, keep the snacks easy-to-digest. Refer to the "Easy vs. Hard to Digest Foods" table in the color insert.

3. **Stop eating nonfood items.** Packaged, processed foods that have an extremely long shelf life do not deserve to be on your plate.

4. **Simplify your meals.** The fewer ingredients, the easier it is to digest. Avoid bad food combinations. More on this in the "Food Combining" chart in the color insert. Try following the Happy Belly meal plan.

5. **Stop eating drying, dehydrating foods.** One of the reasons you get constipated is because you are dehydrated. When your body is dehydrated, your colon is the first to suffer. A healthy colon has a very high percentage of moisture/liquid, and in extreme situations such as dehydration, your body takes liquid from the colon to support other organs. Surprising dehydrating foods are nuts, sandwiches, beans, chips, granola bars, cookies, fiber cereal and bars, undercooked grains, pasta, and bread. Fiber is great, but it needs liquid to move along, so don't forget to drink plenty of pure water.

6. **Soak dried fruit and nuts.** You need to soak them in hot water for at least eight hours. If you're short on time, you can place them in a pot, cover with water, bring to a boil, and then simmer for five minutes (only for dried fruit, not nuts).

7. **Be careful with potatoes, raw apples, celery, popcorn, and puffed cereals.** Generally, white potatoes, raw apples, celery, popcorn, and dry cereal have an astringent quality and may lead to constipation. Red potatoes will be less aggravating, especially if you add coconut oil or ghee. So replace white potatoes with yams or sweet potatoes. If you're having popcorn, add coconut oil or ghee as well. And skip dry cereal all together. Apples and celery can still be eaten but not first thing in the morning on an empty stomach. If constipation is severe, opt for slightly cooked apples. As always, the best way to check if astringent taste constipates you is to experiment: try eating a raw apple or celery on an empty stomach and pay attention if you get bloated and your elimination is influenced.

8. **Hydrate before each meal.** To help the body retain water well, use herbs such as licorice. Hydrating before a meal with a glass of warm water and a wedge of lime/lemon 30 minutes before a meal can be very helpful, according to ayurveda. In between meals, drink a home-made electrolyte drink with a little bit of salt, lime, and honey or raw cane sugar. Soup broths or green smoothies with lime and ginger, cucumber juice, coconut water with cardamom and lime are all great to increase hydration.

9. **Add fiber to your diet slowly.** Oatmeal, well-cooked quinoa, cooked carrots, peas, small lentils, applesauce, greens, and fruit are a great way to start. Do not overload on fiber right away if your gut is not used to it, as it might intensify bloating and constipation even more. Both flaxseeds and chia seeds have very high fiber content. For example, only two tablespoons of flaxseeds and one tablespoon of chia seeds contain about four grams of fiber—as much as one cup of oatmeal. The fibers in

these seeds help add bulk to your stools and will bind on to toxins (including cholesterol) on the way out.

10. **Add some lubricant to the food.** Coconut oil, ghee, and good quality olive oil are great choices. An almond milk chai with coconut oil can help with lubrication to move things along with ease. Don't be afraid of good fats! They are necessary for a healthy digestion and brain function. Plus they keep hunger at bay longer.

11. **Learn to recognize tension and relax it**. Do it by using a warm water bottle on the lower abdomen. Coldness can cause muscle tension. Warmth balances downward-flowing energy and stimulates blood flow to the elimination organs.

12. **Remove coffee** because it can irritate the colon and worsen constipation.

13. **Try anti-spasmatic herbs** to encourage smooth healthy peristalsis—peppermint, lemon balm, cardamom, asafetida, chamomile.

14. **Relax like a pro.** Exhausted people can become constipated; you need rest and relaxation to restore, along with easy-to-digest foods. Download a relaxation guide from www. spinachandyoga.com/resources.

15. **Exercise.** Being sedentary compounds constipation, while even gentle exercise increases the gut's blood flow and improves gastrointestinal motility. Taking a short walk, bouncing around to some good music, or stretching can often help to stimulate elimination. Certain yoga asanas are particularly helpful in

contracting and stretching the abdomen and nudging sluggish systems into gear. You can follow along with me on Happy Belly yoga videos at www.spinachandyoga.com/videos.

16. **Abdominal massage.** Give your belly some love. We take care of our nails, pamper our face, and fuss over our hair, but our internal organs rarely get as much attention. If you've ever been in a managing role, you know that one of the easiest ways to get productive cooperation is to provide rewards and be nice. Similarly, your belly appreciates warmth, love, and attention. Abhyanga, or a general whole-body massage, improves regularity due to its calming effects on the nervous system. A nervous stomach and irritable bowels need some calm and peace. If a whole-body oil massage is an unreachable luxury, try gently rubbing your belly with your palm. Lie on your back, bring your feet into a butterfly (soles of the feet together and knees out to the sides) and gently massage the stomach clockwise. Ayurvedic massage therapists or holistically trained digestive specialists can be of wonderful help.

17. **Breathe deeply.** Take time to breathe and check in with your stomach. If your knees allow it, sit in virasana (ask your yoga teacher if you're unfamiliar with the pose) and do several rounds of deep abdominal breathing. I find it to be a panacea for my digestive troubles. It increases blood flow to the digestive system, while breathing calms your nervous system.

18. **Learn how to sit properly.** Squat or use books or a stool to raise the feet. In a 2003 study, 28 healthy people volunteered to time themselves doing their business in three alternate positions: sitting on a standard toilet, sitting on a low toilet, and

squatting. They not only recorded how long it took them, but also how much effort it took. Squatting, the study concluded, takes less time and effort.[45] "There is definitely some physiologic sense to squatting," says gastroenterologist Anish Sheth, MD, coauthor of the books *What's Your Poo Telling You?* and *What's My Pee Telling Me?*. Simply put, it straightens out the colon. When we're standing, the colon (where waste is stored) gets pushed up against the puborecatlis muscle, which maintains fecal continence until it's time to hit the bathroom. Sitting down only partially relaxes that muscle. Squatting fully relaxes it, essentially straightening out the colon. That, in turn, eases the elimination process. You can order a special step to bring your feet up from Amazon.

19. **Do not suppress the urge to "go." Ever!** The problem with putting off the next bowel movement is that "gastrocolonic response" that creates an urge to "go" may weaken if habitually suppressed. Gastrocolonic response is a neurally mediated increase in high amplitude contractions, which originate in the transverse colon and propagate luminal contents into the sigmoid and the rectum, associated with an urge to defecate. While the stool is sitting in the large intestine, the water from its contents will keep reabsorbing, making your stool drier and drier, which in turn makes it slower and harder to pass.

20. **Learn Agnisar Kriya.** Do it every morning before a meal after having a glass of warm water with lemon. I have been doing it for years and besides strong abs and a flat stomach, it is great for all digestion-related issues. Watch the tutorial here: www. spinachandyoga.com/videos.

21. **Keep a food journal to track which foods or which food combinations trigger the symptoms**. You can download a "Food Log" here: www spinachandyoga.com/resources.

22. **Do a daily visualization** focusing on being regular and eliminating with ease. Use one of the affirmations on page 177 or download a guide to visualization at www.spinachandyoga. com/resources.

chapter 29

DETOX IN AYURVEDA

Detox and cleansing practices are not new. Our ancestors did it, animals in nature do it, and it was traditionally recommended in the ancient text of ayurveda and Chinese medicine. In the past, nature forced us into periods of lighter diet due to the lack of food and poor methods of food preservation. Nowadays, we are responsible for creating a seasonal detox for ourselves.

The goal of the detox is to let our digestive system rest and our body optimize its elimination and detoxification pathways and to nourish our body from the inside out. It helps to support the immune system and efficient digestion, and it prevents disease.

When choosing a cleanse, you have to keep in mind the current state of your health, the result that you are trying to achieve by doing a cleanse, your potential time and effort commitment, your habits around food, eating, and work. You can choose to do three days or 21 days; it is up to you. However, a good number to start with is a simple seven-day cleanse.

A gentle, nourishing seven-day detox will

- let your digestion rest and optimize nutrient absorption.

- help your liver to drive toxins out of your body, making you feel lighter, leaner, and more energized.

- promote elimination through the intestines, kidneys, and skin.

- help you understand your body better and know how to take care of it.

- promote circulation of blood and lymphatic fluid.

- provide you new tools to take care of your body, including healthy recipes, self-massage, detox bath ideas, and health tonics.

- refuel your body with nutrients.

DO YOU NEED TO DETOX?

Regular overeating, indulging in heavy foods, bread, pastries, sweets, and alcohol can create a less-than-ideal state of health. An overburdened digestive system and plugged-up lymphatic system can bring on allergies, sluggishness, water retention, heaviness in the limbs, and seasonal affective disorder.

Anger and persistent depression can even be attributed to an excess of toxins (pesticides and man-made chemicals) in the body. The body gets no pleasure from swimming in its own by-products.

Accumulated undigested food, toxic chemicals from processed products, and a less-than-ideal living environment can negatively affect all aspects of our being, including digestion. If you notice that your tongue is thickly coated in the morning, that joint pain accompanies movement, that your nose feels stuffed even when you don't have a cold, and that even the strongest antiperspirant can't prevent a strong body odor, your body is in dire need of cleansing. Fatigue, mental dullness, irritability, low energy, and lack of inspiration are signs of toxins as well, according to ayurveda.[46]

One of the reasons to declutter and simplify your diet is to increase your sensitivity of your body and perception of the real effect of food on your physical, mental, and emotional state. Your taste buds and your sense of internal well-being become a lot more acute. You notice small shifts that you didn't notice before.

Detox is what you make of it. It can be just a dietary restriction, a regimen with supplements that are supposed to do all the work, or you can turn it into a life-changing restorative experience. I want to share how you can do the latter without fancy pills or difficult recipes to follow — just you, your body, and a few simple practices to help you reconnect and rest.

It is not natural for our bodies to exist on reserve power, to require caffeine to function. A healthy, rested body has plenty of energy throughout the day.

You body can heal faster than anyone wants you to believe. Your job is not to interfere with the process but to allow it to happen. You can foster the change by creating the right environment too.

NO FOOD? NO WAY!

No matter how clogged up, sluggish, and bloated they feel, the idea of having to starve to cleanse is a little scary to most people who can't give up work and family responsibilities and retreat into a week-long cleanse. However, according to ayurveda, detox doesn't have to be scary and stressful. All you need to do is to facilitate and support the natural cleansing process and the organs responsible for it.

Not all cleanses are created equal. Your body is a unique creation with unique needs. Certain cleansing principles will apply to everyone, but a choice between a water fast, juice fast, monomeal cleanse, or elimination diet should be made on an individual basis.

Let's cover general cleansing principles that can be used by everyone first.

DETOX BASICS

The digestive system is just one of the passageways that the body uses to get rid of its byproducts. To make a detox balanced, you need to think of including all bodily systems responsible for naturally cleansing the body. There are several major detox organs in your body: kidneys, colon, skin, liver, and lungs.

A good detox is about simplifying your daily food intake, reducing hard-to-digest foods, and helping your body do its natural work of cleansing. Detox should not be about adding more foods. One important thing to remember is that digestion is a very energy-consuming process. When your body is busy digesting, it has fewer reserves to engage in a full-on detoxification. It does its maintenance cleansing if all the organs function properly, but it is not the same as a deep detox that starts to happen when you reduce the load on digestion.

The less energy spent on digesting food, the more resources your body has to address internal housekeeping such as deep cleansing and healing.

To help your body in the detoxification process, you can add foods, teas, herbs, and supplements that tone the liver, reduce internal inflammation, rebuild healthy gut flora, and help the body expel toxins that are released back into the blood and the digestive tract.

CLEANSE-FACILITATING DIET

The purpose of a cleansing diet is to reduce the workload of the digestive system by providing easy-to-break-down nutrition. The extra energy that will be freed up due to lighter foods can be used by your body to fix and cleanse itself.

- **Some foods can help brush the insides of your stomach and colon** the same way we brush our teeth. Foods that are simple and have a lot of fiber will create a natural intestinal mop to cleanse out all the toxins and mucus that we collected. Think spicy, light, and green! Say no to heavy sauces, everything creamy, or too sweet. A cleanse-facilitating diet means eliminating dairy products, wheat, yeasted breads and other baked goods, fried and oily food, and reducing meat. Instead, meals should be simple and light, composed of berries and fresh, lightly cooked vegetables, grains, and lentils prepared with small amounts of olive oil or ghee, and/or lean protein.

- **A light dinner is crucial to a successful detox program,** since our digestive power weakens considerably in the evening. Simplicity and freshness are a key to any cleanse-friendly diet. Try to eliminate all hard-to-digest foods, and foods that you might be allergic to. For a lot of people it means eliminating wheat, dairy, all processed foods, white sugar, and soy. Try having a green soup or kitchari. Find the recipes in the color insert.

- **Add some bitter greens and spices** to your daily diet to help out a struggling liver. Bitter taste is universally recognized as digestion strengthening. According to Carrie Demers, MD, a board-certified holistic physician, bitter herbs help to detoxify and cool an overworked and overburdened liver while toning the muscles of the digestive tract. They also support detoxification by helping the liver process incoming nutrients and filter impurities from circulation. You can get bitter taste from these herbs: turmeric, dandelion, goldenseal, gentian, milk thistle, and neem. An easy way to add them to your diet is to drink them as tea. Dandelion and milk thistle are my favorite!

- **Drink plenty of liquids.** To stimulate toxin release, try hot water with a pinch of cayenne, one-quarter lemon, one teaspoon of honey, and a few drops of apple cider vinegar. This recipe is recommended by John Immel, the founder of the Joyful Belly website and a great ayurvedic practitioner, as a vivacious ayurvedic blend to boost fat digestion and metabolism. A strong sour taste encourages the free flow of bile from your liver and gall bladder to your gut. This spicy drink restores energy and vitality by helping the body digest high-fat foods. Vinegar and cayenne add an intense metabolic spark that improves energy and enthusiasm. Together with warm water, they strongly stimulate digestion and clear mucus accumulations from the stomach. This has the effect of improving circulation and revving up metabolism. Cumin, coriander, and fennel tea (CCF tea) is cooling and soothing for the mind, the digestion, and the urinary tract. These three kitchen spices are balancing for all seasons and body types. Add one-quarter teaspoon of each spice to two cups of water, bring to the boil, and let it cool. Sip throughout the day.

ELIMINATE THE ENEMY!

All elimination passageways should be optimized to get the best cleansing results. It means that a good cleanse program should always include practices that will help you sweat more, promote regularity, create lymph drainage, and encourage deep breathing.

- **An ayurvedic blend of herbs called triphala can be very helpful**. Triphala is a bowel tonic, not a laxative. It tones the bowel walls and helps the colon function at its optimal level. Ayurvedic texts refer to triphala as a "toxin scraper": it helps pull toxins out of the intestines and draws them out of the body. It is available in most health food stores including Whole Foods.

- **To increase the detoxifying effect, try sauna, steam room, hot baths, and cardio-induced sweating.** Most gyms have sauna and steam rooms that you can use after a workout. If you don't have access to one, take a hot bath with Epsom salt, ginger powder, and baking soda every night before going to sleep. Run, do yoga, jump, dance, whatever gets your heart pumping! Once a week for 20 minutes, sit in a hot bath that contains a handful of Epsom salts, 10 drops of lavender essential oil, and half a cup of baking soda. This combo draws out toxins, lowers stress-related hormones, and balances your pH levels, according to Dr. Mark Hyman, MD.

- **Breathe deeply!** In an always-in-a-rush, stressed-out society, our breath tends to be rushed as well. Our lungs rarely get a chance to breathe fresh—not air-conditioned air—and to cleanse from stale gases. It takes an effort and awareness to let the breath be full and complete. Take a few minutes in the morning to just breathe deeply. Two-to-one breathing—a practice of exhaling twice as long as every inhalation—is a great technique for calming the nervous system and helping your lungs do their job.

SAMPLE DETOX DAILY ROUTINE:

Upon waking up:

- **Scrape your tongue,** brush your teeth, go to the bathroom.
- Drink a large glass of hot water with a thick slice of lemon or lime.
- Take a probiotic and two pills of triphala.
- Make an equal parts **fennel, whole coriander seed, cumin seeds, and fresh ginger tea** by boiling 2 teaspoons in 32 ounces of water for 5–10 minutes and drink it throughout the day from a thermos or at least when you are at home. It has a calming, toning effect on the GI.
- Do some stretching, yoga, or cardio.

Breakfast:

- Try millet with one date and hemp seeds, or quinoa with diced vegetables, buckwheat, or kitchari. Breakfast katchari recipe variations are in the color insert.

- A slightly stewed apple with three prunes and three apricots, nutmeg, and cloves can be a great breakfast too. Follow with 10–15 soaked and peeled almonds.

- Sip nettle, mint, or coriander, cumin, fennel tea. Or any tea from the recipes from the previous chapter.

Snack:

- Berries, low glycemic fruit, or avocado with sea salt, black pepper and lime juice.

- Sip more hot herbal tea.

Lunch:

- Your biggest meal: Focus on veggies, legumes and some whole grains such as quinoa or veggies and lean protein.

- Some ideas: lentil soup with roasted or steamed veggies. Kitchari with a side of greens. Recipes are in the color insert.

- Wild salmon with steamed vegetables and a side salad. Try adding a green soup to some meals (recipe: www.spinachandyoga.com/recipes and in the color insert).

Predinner:

- Bath soak with Epsom salt, ginger, and baking soda.

Dinner:

- Keep it light with soup, veggie curry, kitchari or fish.

- Sip more tea.

Before bedtime:

- Take triphala.

- Gratitude journal: list three things that you did well for your body today and things that you are grateful for. Keep them unique to today.

- Guided relaxation before sleep. Try the ones at www.spinachandyoga.com/resources.

Note: refer to the meal plan in the photo section.

Bonus Tips

- Avoid eating leftovers, processed foods, and foods grown with chemical fertilizers and pesticides. Your body has to work that much harder to eliminate the impurities found in these foods.

- Avoid cold drinks, which reduce the digestive fire and result in the formation of digestive toxins known as ama in ayurveda.

- Drink plenty of warm water throughout the day to flush out impurities. Make sure your water is filtered to remove environmental toxins.

- Avoid exposure to cigarette smoke, alcohol, drugs, chemicals, environmental pollution, and other toxins.

- Go to bed by 10 p.m. so your body can rest during its natural purification cycle, from 10 p.m. to 2 a.m.

- Do a yoga nidra or another type of daily deep relaxation.

- Get a massage.

- Get good-quality sleep.

- Stretch often.

- Reduce bright screen time (TV and computer).

- Before bedtime, write in your gratitude journal.

During the first few days after giving up customary foods, caffeine, and sugar, you might experience some withdrawal symptoms such as fatigue, headache, and cravings, but these won't last forever. In a few days your body will start feeling better: revived, light, and energetic.

Here is what you are looking to get with a good cleanse:

- better sleep.

- great energy throughout the day without ups and downs.

- a less sluggish feeling in the morning.

- clear, glowing skin.

- improved digestion.

- peaceful, clear mind and inspiration.

- increased comfort in your body.

JUICING IN AYURVEDA

Juice cleanses are everywhere! Every celebrity is doing them and every other deli claims to have a juice bar. There are companies that will deliver juices to your door every morning. All the marketing, skinny, hip-looking people publicly sipping green liquid, and a huge celebrity following probably make you wonder if drinking a green-monster concoction will set you free from extra baggage sticking around and heal your digestion.

A few years ago I was an ardent juicer myself. I would drink juices every day and drink just green juice with no food once a week: two to three quarts of green juice with lemon and ginger (no apples, carrots, or beets—just greens) and nothing else. This was my way of letting my digestive system rest from solid food and detox, or so I thought.

In August 2010, I met Dr. Vasant Lad and my pretty green world turned upside down. During a two-day ayurvedic workshop on ayurvedic diagnostic techniques, I received unexpected explanations for my occasional digestion issues, fatigue, and constantly cold hands. When Dr. Lad matter-of-factly noted that my weekly juices were to blame and suggested I boil my precious, enzyme-rich vegetables before juicing, I couldn't believe what I heard! It didn't make any sense!

But Dr. Lad had a wisdom I was just beginning to tap into. So the research started—and still continues to this day. Here is what I have found so far and **how you can use it to get the most out of your juice cleanse if you decide to do it.**

- **Juice cleansing is not for everyone, but everyone can benefit from some mild green juices.** All the advice in ayurveda depends on who we are talking about. Body constitution, eating habits, current lifestyle, and the time of the year have to be considered before embarking on any kind of a cleanse. Cleansing in general can be good because your stomach will have more time to digest leftover food and spend time on self-healing. Potentially, it can give more energy and lightness to the body and mind.

    Different body constitutions can benefit from different cleansing methods. One can try eating light foods, eating

304

just fruits, skipping one meal, skipping food for the entire day, going on juices for a day, drinking just water or herbal tea.

Vata-types: Juice cleanses are not recommended for vata-type people because, due to their weak digestive system, raw juices will make them bloated and tired. If you are a pure vata type or have been experiencing any digestive issues lately, start by eating light meals at regular times of the day. Vata types also can do slightly warmed juices made with vata-appropriate vegetables and fruit such as fennel, ginger, pears, and pineapple.

Pitta-predominant types can't tolerate complete fasting because their metabolism is very strong. Juice fasting with cooling and blood purifying vegetables is a good option for pitta types.

Kaphas are ideal people for fasting. They can skip one meal or go on a regimen of no food for an entire day. Kapha types will feel full of energy on juice cleanses.

- **Juice is a superconcentrated food.** And it requires chewing! How long would it take you to chew the five pounds of greens that go into a glass of juice? Often we gulp it down the same way as water without paying attention to taste. Sip your juice slowly and let your body process the taste and the effects of a super-concentrated elixir. Chewing and tasting food is beneficial for digestion and lets your body recognize all the nutrients. Make juice drinking an exercise of mindfulness!

- **Juice doesn't last for three days!** Juice loses its precious qualities pretty quickly. As soon as a fruit or vegetable is processed, the natural enzymes in the juice begin to break down the other nutrients. Because vegetables contain more enzymes than fruits, their nutrients are depleted faster. "Once vegetable juices start to thicken, all that's left are water, minerals and calories," says Dr. Steven Bailey, ND, a naturopathic physician. It is best to drink your juice within 30 minutes.

- **Bloating and fatigue are to be expected in the first couple of days.** As soon as you restrict food intake, your body turns to other pressing responsibilities instead of digestion. Quite often it will be cleaning out byproducts and undigested food leftovers and healing. This can leave you feeling tired and sleepy, especially on the second or third day of juice fasting. If you decide to do a juice fast, choose a period of time when you can cut down on physical and mental activity and let your body rest and restore.

- **Be strategic about what goes into your juice.** Different fruits and vegetables have different effects on our body. While some are stimulating the detoxification process on the cellular level, others are just pleasant-tasting fructose. Do your research and ask for a specific mixture at the juice bar. A great combo for a sensitive digestion is cucumber, fennel, mint, and lime. In the cold months you can experiment with adding some beet, carrot, kale, and lemon juice as these ingredients are particularly effective at stimulating the liver and warming. Carrots help fight seasonal mood slumps and brighten up the skin. Ayurveda also recommends adding some spices to boost the effects of juices and making them less vata-aggravating. Good juice additions are ginger, black pepper, aloe vera gel, and curcumin (turmeric). Curcumin, for example, has been shown to prevent and/or cure cancer in laboratory tests.[47] Turmeric is also used to support liver function. It acts as anti-inflammatory, purifies the body, creates glowing skin, and can aid in indigestion and gallstones. Dr. Andrew Weil, founder and director of the Arizona Center for Integrative Medicine, notes that turmeric also helps balance cholesterol levels and boosts the immunity system, and modern research has found it beneficial in the treatment of Alzheimer's. Try it in a carrot juice!

- **Juice is not enough to cleanse.** Actually, it can easily cause bloating and irregularity. Traditionally, an important part of juice fasting was the use of laxatives or enemas to cleanse the lower digestive tract because the juice will not supply enough fiber to keep the bowels moving. Since the removal of wastes is essential to prevent the toxins in the digestive tract from being reabsorbed into the bloodstream, juicing professionals recommend mixtures of slippery elm or other herbs to cleanse the bowels while on the juice-only fast. Triphala can also help.

- **Juice doesn't substitute for real vegetables.** Most people on the standard American diet (SAD) are commonly lacking fiber. So drink your juice all you want, but make sure to eat fresh vegetables to keep your body clean throughout the whole year.

···

chapter 30

HAPPY HEALTHY PARTIES AND AFTER-PARTIES

O ften our friends and family might be less healthy in their routines, especially those related to food. Once you know how feeling healthy, light, and easy in your body feels, it is not easy to go back to feeling heavy, sluggish, and bloated.

Family dinners cause a lot of stress and anxiety in many health warriors who are striving their best to protect their health and digestion day to day. Many of my clients have said that they feel tension building in their body when they imagine sitting at a family table and having to explain why they refuse gravy or take just one cookie instead of loading their plate along with everyone else.

Some of us might also feel fear because we are not sure of our ability to resist temptation and say no. We are afraid of regaining the weight that we worked so hard to get rid of. The universe works in such a way that whatever you focus on tends to happen. So if you focus on things that you are afraid of, or things that you are not looking forward to, they will come into your life.

If your body fills up with resistance and you get an influx of negative emotions thinking about an upcoming food combination, I have a few useful tips for you. First, remember that whatever happened in the past doesn't have to happen again. You build your life a day at time. You are in full control when it comes to the outcome of a family dinner. You can even shift the way everyone feels if you choose to.

Actionable and Effective Tips To Stay Healthy During The Holidays

1. Remember, your body is not your enemy; it is your only lifelong partner. She deserves love and respect. She deserves celebration, beautiful food made with love, not fast food. She deserves to have fun.

2. If you are not eating certain foods due to a food sensitivity, don't think of it as restricting food. Instead, think of it as preserving energy that would go to digesting difficult foods for healing. The food that you might be craving will be there later when your digestive system is healed.

3. Pay attention to how you think about the upcoming party or dinner. Are you dreading a meal? Are you afraid that you won't be full after it? Are you scared that your willpower is not strong enough? At one point I caught myself thinking: "Am I going to get enough protein, enough greens? Will it be cooked properly? Are there still enzymes left? Is it going to make me bloated?" I was almost scared of food. I treated it with so much calculation that the pleasure of eating was gone. It was more like a math class. And no one likes math three times a day! Choose to love your food and the food will be more likely to leave your body feeling good.

Before the party:

- **Keep your diet simple and light the day before the feast.** Our digestive power is like any other muscle: it works better after a rest period. If you push yourself really hard one day, you will have less muscle strength available to you the next day. Marathoners don't run the day before the marathon to save up the energy before a major push. Have a light meal the day before the party so your digestion is strong the day of. A light meal day does not mean that you have to starve yourself. It means sticking to easy-to-digest foods and simple food combinations. A sample light day can be: oatmeal or a smoothie for breakfast, lentil soup or salmon with a little bit of quinoa and a side of greens for lunch, a baked apple or berries for a snack, and a vegetable stew or a soup for dinner.

- **Encourage family members and friends to set up early dinners or better yet, lunches!** The earlier you eat, the more time your body will have to digest the food. Our digestion is the strongest during the daytime but gets weak and sluggish after sundown.

- **Bring a healthy dish if the party is at someone's house.** Be an example for others and provide a fall-back dish for yourself. Roasted vegetables and butternut squash side dishes are perfect examples.

- **Visualize how you want to feel and behave around food.** I imagine myself feeling nourished, relaxed, and grateful in front of the table.

At the party:

- **Drink a glass of warm water 20 minutes before a meal.** It can improve digestive function by as much as **24 percent** because warm water will increase the blood flow to the stomach. The better your digestion, the less likely you are to feel heavy and sleepy after a meal.

- **Avoid cold drinks with your food.** Cold drinks contract blood vessels and reduce the blood flow to the stomach, which is damaging to healthy digestion.

- **Get your heart rate up before sitting down to eat.** Throw your little niece or nephew up in the air a few times (they'll love it), do 50 jumping jacks and squats before the meal. Ayurvedically speaking, the exercise will kindle your digestive fire and prepare your body to digest a meal. Tim Ferris of *The 4-Hour Body* swears by this technique.

- **Be an inspiring role model.** Don't lecture or look down upon anyone not following your rules. The only way to create change is by inspiring people to experiment and explore new ways; it is never done through coercion.

- **Sprinkle sweets and cake with cinnamon.**

- **Chew every bite and don't compete with others on cleaning up your plate first.** Focus on enjoying the flavors, colors, and the smell of food. Stay mindful of how you feel and how full your stomach is!

- **Enjoy the connection with other people, not just the food.** Make social events about being social. When you are absorbed in an exciting conversation, it will be a lot easier to ignore the greasy food.

After the party:

- **Relax for 15 minutes after the food and then move.** John Immel, the founder of a great ayurvedic website, *Joyful Belly*, advises to guard your digestion and relax after eating. He says that after eating, blood rushes to the stomach to supply stomach glands with fluids. The food is mixed with acids and slowly digests. About 15 minutes after eating, the food is fully hydrated and the flow of blood to the stomach relaxes somewhat. To ensure a proper supply of blood, rest at least 15 minutes after eating. Avoid any strenuous exercise or difficult mental tasks, such as studying, for two hours after eating.

- **Sip detoxifying, magical ginger tea.** Freshly steeped ginger tea with lemon will help settle your stomach. If there is no way to get a fresh ginger root, take a few ginger tea packets with you to the party. Pukka teas and Gaia herbs have a huge selection of detox and digestion stimulating teas. Don't forget to share them with your suffering friends!

- **Help your natural detoxification mechanism.** If you notice any signs of indigestion such as gas, bloating, burping, acid reflux, constipation, and feeling tired after eating, it means that you overloaded your stomach. Be kind to yourself and help the natural detoxification processes. Triphala is a wonderful, age-proven, science-supported bowel tonic. It is not a laxative like many over-the-counter detox packs. It is popular in ayurveda due to its unique ability to gently cleanse and detoxify the system while simultaneously replenishing and nourishing it. This traditional formula supports the proper functions of the digestive, circulatory, respiratory and genitourinary systems. Tea can be another good option—a mixture of licorice root, cardamom seed, fennel, coriander, ginger, and black pepper will alleviate indigestion and reduce heavy feelings in the stomach

Make it a light meal day the next day if your stomach is still not back to normal. Signs that your body is back to normal: healthy pink tongue, no swelling on your face and fingers, no heavy feeling in the stomach, and a true hunger.

A DIFFICULT CHOICE

As a beginning wellness warrior, you face a difficult choice: your health and balance versus your relationship with old friends. On long weekends when most people get together to celebrate, relaxing and "having fun" can be particularly challenging. You don't want to seem "boring" and "weird." You want to feel a part of the group, relax, and have fun too. Most of your friends may still be not sold on all the aspects of a healthy lifestyle. They may consider early dinners an entertainment for grandpas, and they may love to dance into the wee hours. The good thing is that if you know how to rebalance yourself, you and your digestion will recover a lot quicker.

Those of you who think that being healthy is too boring and overrated and fear missing the next big DJ a lot more than damaging your liver and hurting your tummy, you might pick up a few useful tips from this section. Trust me. You don't need to turn into a health nut right away, but being kinder to your body a few days a week will make your off-party days so much happier.

Clean Body = Sensitive Body

It feels amazing to live in a clean, healthy body that has a lot of energy and mind clarity. Once experienced, this state is not something one would want to give up easily!

Sadly, a clean body reacts a lot more strongly to pollutants such as alcohol, bad food, or recreational drugs. It becomes more sensitive. As a result, I often hear from my clients that after not drinking any alcohol for a month, they feel sick after one glass of wine. I experienced it myself, and it is not pleasant. It makes perfect sense, however. How would a kid feel if you give him alcohol? Probably pretty sick too. Once your body is clean, it doesn't tolerate toxic substances and has a healthy reaction of wanting to eliminate the toxins as fast as possible.

Peer pressure, and lack of desire to be the "weird" one and completely break away from an old group of friends usually leads to giving up some of the daily health rules for a night or two. Not ideal but not the end of the world!

If you feel crappy, tired, and bloated the next day, there are a few things that you can do to restore balance. We'll focus on physical and mental/emotional aspects equally. You are a whole being and you need to balance out all aspects.

Physical ER

Being out really late, in a loud place, surrounded by a lot of people, drinking, smoking, and doing any kind of drug creates a major imbalance in a lot of systems. Hormones, blood chemistry, stomach lining, water levels, digestion, liver, kidney, pancreas (alcohol is a highly concentrated sugar), nervous system—your entire body and mind become slightly or extremely out of whack.

There are many common-sense practices that help to restore the physical body back to balance. To find out what will work the best for your body, ask it what it needs to recover. If you are attentive enough, you will know intuitively what to do. Most likely, your body needs a combination of hydrating drinks, sleep, gentle stretching, and nourishing food. Stretching and easy-to-digest food are crucial to restore energy and to break up stiff points of tension. Here is a list of tips that have worked really well for me and a few of my friends.

- **Drink a glass or two of warm water with lemon or lime** first thing in the morning.

- **Drink coconut water** before breakfast or lunch. Alcohol, smoking, greasy/heavy food, and dancing until early morning creates a lot of heat in the body. Cool coconut helps to calm it down while rehydrating your thirsty body. Potassium and electrolytes help.

- **Eat simple meals throughout the day.** To restore energy and let your liver and digestion recuperate, use fewer ingredients and let simplicity rule. This will ensure that your meals are easy to digest (less likelihood of bad food combinations) and won't overtax your digestive system. Congee, kitchari, and vegetable soup with simple protein are great choices if you are up for cooking. If you are eating out or ordering in, try vegetable soups, a light curry, stir-fries, baked salmon, or plain quinoa with greens.

- **Do a Yoga Nidra.** Deep restorative rest for the entire system helps to get back to a normal level of energy a lot faster than just melting in front of the TV. You can download a yoga nidra recording at www.spinachandyoga. com/resources.

- **Go for a walk outside.** Breaking up the routine and staying up all night is a big stress for the body, whether you realize it or not. To regulate natural cycles and to get back to a routine, sunlight and fresh air are great helpers. Take a short walk during your lunchtime or after work.

Mental and Emotional ER

You need to know and believe that the *real you* is still happy, perfect, and full of light. It is your body and your mind that feels tired and depressed. Once you realize that you are unchangeable, constant, and always happy, it is a lot easier to deal with a body and mind that are experiencing the consequences of weekend-long abuse.

The goal of the guidelines below is to create a positive state of mind and get out of a depressing mood.

- **Let go of the guilt.** What's done is done, no point in fussing over it. Focus on what you can do to make yourself feel better in the present instead of thinking about what you should've done differently the day before. Now is the only thing that matters. Learning to let go will save you a lot of negative emotions.

- **List things you are grateful for** and that are still going great even though you feel crappy. Keep doing it throughout the day, especially when an overwhelming desire to complain and to feel sorry for yourself appears.

- **Visualize** energy coming in and fatigue and toxins going out with every breath. Close your eyes and play with your imagination

- **Smile, listen to good music, call happy friends**, do whatever you need to do to get out of a negative state and create positive, happy thoughts. Remember that the outside is just a reflection of what's inside.

final words

Now that you are done reading this book, you have a lot of tips to experiment with. Hopefully, you understand your body better and feel empowered with new knowledge.

I would like to bring something interesting to your attention, something that I have thought about for years and that several of my teachers helped me solidify.

Once we learn something, we cannot give it back. We can choose not to accept that knowledge or not to believe it. But if that knowledge is true and we know deep in our heart that it is true, it becomes a part of our wisdom.

For example: a wisdom that I know is true because I lived through it is that eating in a peaceful, calm environment and mindfully chewing my food leaves me feeling light and easy after a meal and prevents overeating. I know that this is true. I believe it with all my heart and my gut. However, I don't always do it.

My friend, ayurvedic chef Divya Alter, said, "We are punished with indigestion and bloating, not only for eating fast with a phone in our hand, but we are also punished mentally for ignoring our body's wisdom. We experience guilt. We feel that we failed ourselves. What it comes down to is that we don't feel that we can trust ourselves, that we can't live in integrity with our body."

Those who don't possess this wisdom can still be punished but not as much. They won't have as much emotional and mental negativity. Theirs will be mostly physical.

It takes strength to live in integrity with your body's wisdom. You become the carrier of knowledge and responsible for implementing it. However, honing your body's wisdom and respecting it can create a sense of empowerment and finally, an ability to bring your body back into balance.

I hope you will be a proud carrier of this knowledge, someone who lives in accordance with her wisdom. I am still working on it and can share that it is an incredibly interesting journey.

One of my friends and clients gave me great advice a few days before the manuscript of this book was due at the publisher. She asked me if the book was easy to absorb and not too overwhelming.

We have covered a lot of topics, and there is still a lot left to discuss. We are complicated and intricate creatures. But fortunately, the biggest shift is usually achieved with simple changes.

So, below, I want to summarize a few main take-aways that in my opinion can make a big difference to anyone's digestion if applied on a daily basis.

When you think of improving your digestion, getting rid of bloating and getting regular, there are two things to keep in mind. One is that, regardless of your symptoms, it is a matter of soothing the irritation by taking away all aggravating foods and using supplements and herbs to allow healing to happen. The other important point to remember is that you should analyze your food/eating to discover what brought on the symptoms to begin with. Food sensitivities, leaky gut, bloating, and constipation are all symptoms that reflect an imbalance due to habits, diet, or lifestyle. If that initial reason is not addressed, the symptoms will keep coming back.

Here are my final words to your belly and to you:

- Write out your wellness vision and come back to it every single day. Meditate on it, connect with it, and become it.

- Eat to balance your body (sluggish to light, constipated to regular). Learn to understand the "like increases like and opposites balance" concept and apply it to help your body.

- Focus on easy-to-digest foods 80 percent of the time and allow for some flexibility in the remaining 20 percent.

- Give your digestion time—no constant munching.

- Use healing spices.

- Drink teas—keep your belly warm.

- Let your belly rest from time to time with monomeals and seasonal detox.

- When feeling sluggish, constipated, and bloated, focus on eating only easy-to-digest, very simple food. Limit hard-to-digest, multiple-ingredient dishes—eat plain, simple, and light bland until your stomach feels better.

- No fruit after meals.

- Stretch and engage your core.

- Breathe into your belly and don't be afraid to touch it and even massage it with love.

- Eat your biggest meal when you are relaxed. When stressed and tired, choose to focus on light and liquid foods.

- Eat fresh, whole food and avoid processed and packaged food.

- Eat what makes your body feel best and avoid trigger foods.

- Include an abundance of fiber in your diet from fresh fruits, vegetables, and whole, unprocessed grains.

Be kind to your body—you are on one team!

For a complete list of helpful resources, visit www.spinachandyoga.com/resources.

notes and bibliography

1 National Digestive Diseases Information Clearinghouse (NDDIC), "Digestive Diseases Statistics for the United States," accessed June 27, 2013, http://digestive.niddk.nih.gov/statistics/statistics.aspx.

2 Ibid.

3 Alexandro Junger, *Clean—Expanded Edition: The Revolutionary Program to Restore the Body's Natural Ability to Heal Itself* (New York: HarperCollins, 2009).

4 Alexandro Junger, "Root Cause of Disease," in *Clean Gut: The Breakthrough Plan for Eliminating the Root Cause of Disease and Revolutionizing Your Health* (New York: HarperCollins, 2013), 1–11.

5 Mark Hyman, *The UltraMind Solution: Fix Your Broken Brain by Healing Your Body First: The Simple Way to Defeat Depression, Overcome Anxiety, and Sharpen Your Mind* (New York: Simon & Schuster, 2008).

6 Shirley S. Wang, "A Gut Check for Many Ailments," *Wall Street Journal,* WSJ.com, accessed June 27, 2013, http://on.wsj.com/ypFCjI.

7 Ibid.

8 Ibid.

9 Adam Hadhazy, "Think Twice: How the Gut's 'Second Brain' Influences Mood and Well-Being," *Scientific American*, accessed June 27, 2013, http://www.scientificamerican.com/article/gut-second-brain/.

10 Pamela Popper and Glen Merzer, "Diseases and the Foods That Bring Them On," in *Food over Medicine: The Conversation That Could Save Your Life* (Dallas: Benbella, 2013), 45–93.

11 The Ayurvedic Institute, Home page, accessed June 27, 2013, http://www.ayurveda.com/.

12 Walter Kacera, *Ayurvedic Tongue Diagnosis* (Twin Lakes, Wisconsin: Lotus Press, 2006).

13 Deepak Chopra, *Perfect Digestion: The Key to Balanced Living* (New York: Harmony Books, 1995).

14 "Agricultural Fact Book," U.S. Department of Agriculture, accessed June 27, 2013, http://www.usda.gov/documents/usda-factbook-2001-2002.pdf.

15 Kathleen Zelman, "The Hidden Ingredient That Can Sabotage Your Diet," MedicineNet.com, accessed May 1, 2013, http://www.medicinenet.com/script/main/art.asp?articlekey=56589.

16 "Americans' Ton-a-Year Eating Habit: By the Numbers," *The Week*, Jan. 2, 2012, accessed Aug. 1, 2013, http://theweek.com/article/index/222922/americans-ton-a-year-eating-habit-by-the-numbers.

17 Charlie Donham, "Interview with Aajonus Vonderplanitz," *Natural Health M2M*, October 1, 1998, available on Dr. Stanley Bass's website at http://www.drbass.com/aajonus.html

18 John Douillard, "Digestive Enzymes—the Hidden Dangers," *Life Spa*, Sept. 26, 2012, accessed December 28, 2012, http://www.lifespa.com/digestive-enzymes-the-hidden-dangers/.

19 Lissa Rankin, *Mind over Medicine: Scientific Proof That You Can Heal Yourself* (Carlsbad: Hay House, 2013).

20 National Digestive Diseases Information Clearinghouse (NDDIC), "Digestive Diseases Statistics," accessed June 2013, http://digestive.niddk.nih.gov/ddiseases/pubs/constipation/.

21 P. J. Boekema, M. Samsom, G. P. van Berge Henegouwen, and A. J. Smout, "Coffee and Gastrointestinal Function: Facts and Fiction, a Review," *Scandinavian Journal of Gastroenterology*, Supplement 230 (1999): 35–39.

22 Rajneesh Kumar Sharma, MD, "On the Effects of Coffee, 1803, Dr. Samuel Hahnemann" *Homeopathy World Community* (blog), July 16, 2010, accessed June 27, 2013, http://www.homeopathyworldcommunity.com/profiles/blogs/on-the-effects-of-coffee-1803.

23 Ibid.

24 J. Visser, J. Rozing, A. Sapone, K. Lammers, and A. Fasano, "Tight Junctions, Intestinal Permeability," *Annals of the New York Academy of Science*, May 2009, accessed June 28, 2013, http://www.ncbi.nlm.nih.gov/pubmed/19538307.

25 Joe Rubino, *Dream Manifesto* (blog) accessed June 28, 2013, http://www.dreammanifesto.com/create-vision-life.html.

26 Rankin, *Mind Over Medicine.*

27 Claudia Welch, *Balance Your Hormones, Balance Your Life: Achieving Optimal Health and Wellness Through Ayurveda, Chinese medicine, and Western Science* (Cambridge, Massachusetts: Da Capo Lifelong, 2011).

28 "Paul Brunton Philosophic Foundation – "NOTEBOOKS & IDEAS," accessed June 28, 2013, http://www.paulbrunton.org/notebooksandideas.php.

29 Herbert Benson, *The Relaxation Response* (New York: Morrow, 1975).

30 Herbert Benson, "Stress Management: Approaches for Preventing and Reducing Stress," *Harvard Health Publications*, n.d., accessed Aug. 4, 2013, http://www.health.harvard.edu/special_health_reports/stress-management-approaches-for-preventing-and-reducing-stress.

31 K. J. Sherman, E. J. Ludman, A. J. Cook, R. J. Hawkes, P. P. Roy-Byrne, S. Bentley, M. Z. Brooks, and D. C. Cherkin (2010), "Effectiveness of Therapeutic Massage for Generalized Anxiety Disorder: A Randomized Controlled Trial," *Depression and Anxiety* 27 (2010): 441–450, doi: 10.1002/da.20671.

32 "Mindfulness: The Unconventional Research of Psychologist Ellen Langer," *Harvard Magazine*, Sept.-Oct. 2010, accessed June 28, 2013, http://harvard-magazine.com/2010/09/the-mindfulness-chronicles.

33 Stewart Wolf, "The Effects of Suggestion and Conditioning on the Action of Chemical Agents in Human Subjects: The Pharmacology of Placebos," *Journal of Clinical Investigation* 29, no. 1 (January 1950): 100–109.

34 Henry K. Beecher, "The Powerful Placebo," *Journal of the American Medical Association* 159, no. 17 (December 24, 1955): 1602–6.

35 Stanley Bass, "Self Mastery through Attentive Eating," *Dr. Stanley S. Bass: Super Nutrition & Superior Health* (blog), accessed June 28, 2013, http://www.drbass.com/attentive.html.

36 Stanley Bass, "Sequential Eating & Food Combining: Correct Food Combinations," *Dr. Stanley S. Bass: Super Nutrition & Superior Health* (blog), accessed June 28, 2013, http://www.drbass.com/sequential.html.

37 Richard Wiseman, *59 Seconds: Think a Little, Change a Lot* (New York: Knopf, 2009).

38 Leo Babauta, "The Little Book of Contentment," *Zen Habits* (blog), accessed June 28, 2013, http://zenhabits.net/little-book/.

39 Sasha T. Loring, *Eating with Fierce Kindness: A Mindful and Compassionate Guide to Losing Weight* (Oakland, California: New Harbinger, 2010).

40 Thomas Yarema and Daniel Rhoda, *Eat-Taste-Heal: An Ayurvedic Cookbook of Modern Living* (Kapaa, Hawaii: Five Elements, 2006).

41 "Effect of Food on Temperament," *Ayurveda for You* (blog), accessed Oct. 20, 2013, http://ayurveda-foryou.com/treat/foodtemparament.html.

42 Maharishi ayurveda, the preeminent system of herbal medicine, health supplements, ayurvedic products, herbal remedies and herbal supplements, Maharishi Ayurveda Products International, accessed Oct. 20, 2013, http://www.mapi.com/maharishi_ayurveda/products/ayurveda_herbal_remedies/vatatea.html.

43 Heather Van Vorous, "Organic Peppermint Tummy Tea for IBS pain and Irritable Bowel Syndrome spasms and cramps," Help for IBS.com (irritable bowel treatments, diet, and IBS education), accessed Oct. 20, 2013, http://www.helpforibs.com/teas/peppermint.asp.

44 Katherine Czapp, "Putting Polish on Those Humble Beans," Weston A. Price Foundation ("For Wise Traditions in Food, Farming, and the Healing Arts"), accessed February 24, 2012, http://www.westonaprice.org/food-features/putting-the-polish-on-those-humble-beans.

45 J. Dalessio, "Are You Pooping Wrong?" *Everyday Health* (blog), accessed October 20, 2013, http://www.everydayhealth.com/digestive-health/are-you-pooping-wrong.aspx.

46 Shannon Sexton, "What Can Panchakarma Do for You?" *Yoga International*, May 20, 2013, accessed Oct. 21, 2013, http:// yogainternational.com/ article/view/what-can-panchakarma-do-for-you.

47 "Specific Foods, Herbs, and Spices That May Help Fight Cancer and Reduce Treatment Side Effects," *Meals to Heal*, accessed Oct. 21, 2013, http://meals-to-heal.com/nutritional-resources/specific-foods-herbs-and-spices/.

··

NADYA ANDREEVA is a certified wellness coach professionally trained in mindful eating and yoga. Nadya's mission is to support women in reconnecting to their bodies and creating a trusting mind-body relationship. Through mindfulness, the ancient wisdom of ayurveda, and positive psychology, Nadya helps her clients to live in alignment between desires and action to achieve their personal image of best self. She holds an MA in organizational psychology from New York University and she is a certified health and wellness coach of the Wellcoaches School of Coaching, endorsed by the American College of Sports Medicine (ACSM). Nadya has also completed residential training in yoga and vedanta, anatomy for yoga teachers, and multiple workshops on ayurveda.

www.spinachandyoga.com

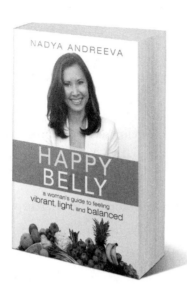

How can you use this book?

MOTIVATE

EDUCATE

THANK

INSPIRE

PROMOTE

CONNECT

Why have a custom version of *Happy Belly*?

- Build personal bonds with customers, prospects, employees, donors, and key constituencies
- Develop a long-lasting reminder of your event, milestone, or celebration
- Provide a keepsake that inspires change in behavior and change in lives
- Deliver the ultimate "thank you" gift that remains on coffee tables and bookshelves
- Generate the "wow" factor

Books are thoughtful gifts that provide a genuine sentiment that other promotional items cannot express. They promote employee discussions and interaction, reinforce an event's meaning or location, and they make a lasting impression. Use your book to say "Thank You" and show people that you care.